SpringerBriefs in Bioengineering

More information about this series at http://www.springer.com/series/10280

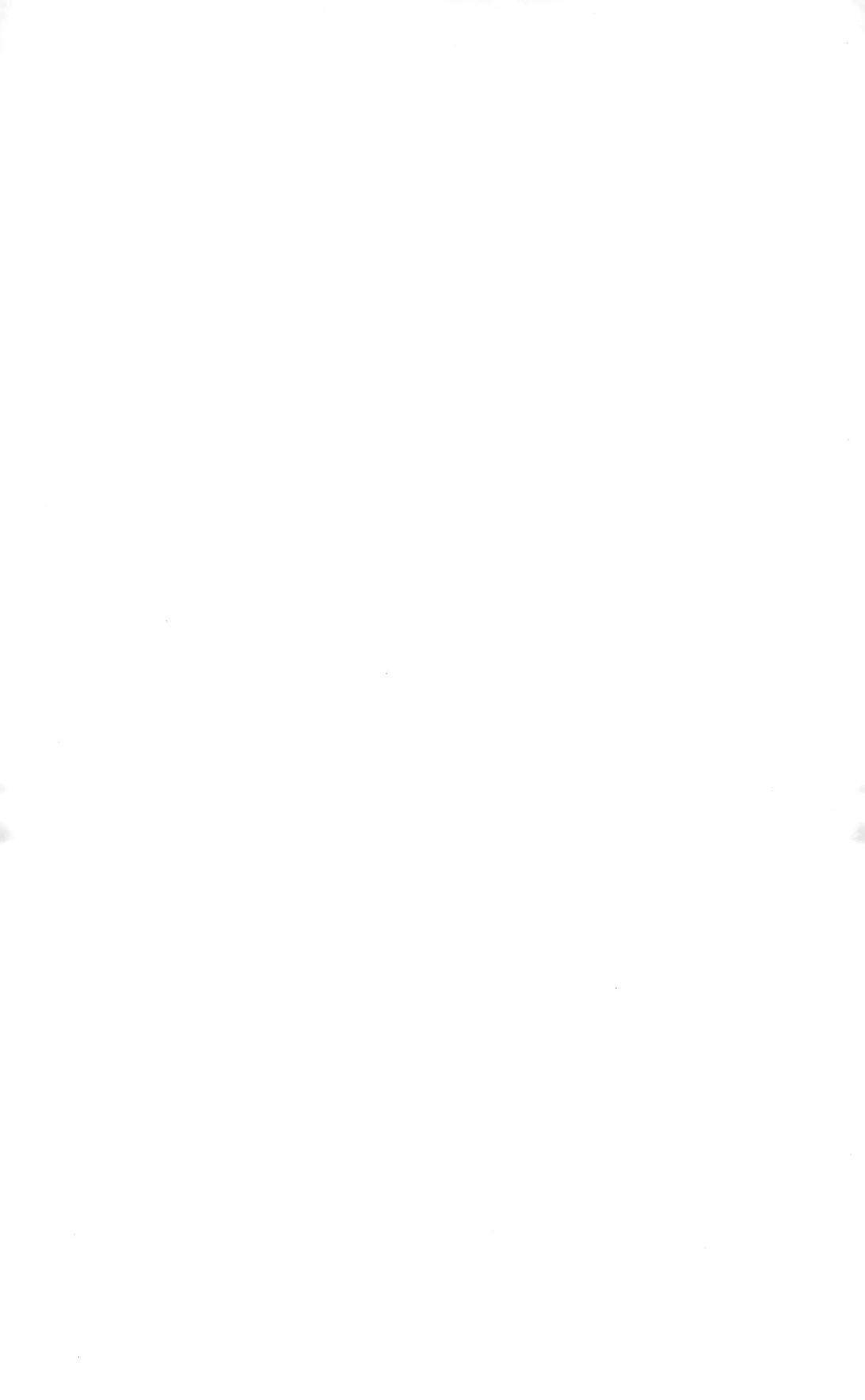

Pogaku Ravindra • Kenthorai Raman Jegannathan

Production of biodiesel using lipase encapsulated in κ-carrageenan

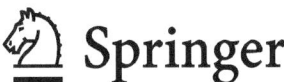 Springer

Pogaku Ravindra
University Malaysia Sabah School
  of Engineering & Info tech
Kota Kinabalu, Malaysia

Kenthorai Raman Jegannathan
École polytechnique fédérale de Lausanne
Lausanne, Switzerland

ISSN 2193-097X   ISSN 2193-0988 (electronic)
ISBN 978-3-319-10821-6 ISBN 978-3-319-10822-3 (eBook)
DOI 10.1007/978-3-319-10822-3
Springer Cham Heidelberg New York Dordrecht London

Library of Congress Control Number: 2014952902

Printed on acid-free paper

Springer is part of Springer Science+Business Media (www.springer.com)

Dedicated to my dazzling grand daughter "Medhanwitha" who inspired me to delve deep into sustainable energy for future generations

Contents

Chapter 1
Introduction

Abstract The introduction covers the need for biofuels along with their types, global biodiesel production details and the history of biodiesel. The history of palm oil, the palm oil market trends and the need for biodiesel production in Malaysia are also discussed. The biodiesel companies in Malaysia, the current biodiesel technology and the need for research in sustainable technology, lipase enzyme and polymer material and their advantages and application are reported. In addition, the overall objectives and the specific objectives of this research work are also presented.

The availability and environmental impact of energy resources will play a critical role in the progress of the world's societies and the physical future of our planet. Worldwide energy consumption is increasing exponentially (Fig. 1.1) and at present usage rates, these sources will soon be exhausted (Srivastava and Prasad 2000), contributed to soaring fossil fuel prices. The majority of human energy needs are currently met using petrochemical sources, coal and natural gases. As the demand for energy has grown, so have the adverse environmental effects of its production.

Emissions of CO_2 (Fig. 1.2), SO_2 and NO_x from fossil fuel combustion are the primary causes of adverse environmental effects (Ture et al. 1997). The accumulation of carbon dioxide and other greenhouse gases in the atmosphere is thought to be responsible for climate change, which is predicted to have disastrous global consequences for life on this planet (Sheehan et al. 1998). Renewable energy may offer an excellent alternative to the fossil fuels, representing a cornerstone to steer our energy system in the direction of sustainability and supply security. Hence, Renewable energy sources have become a high priority in the energy policy strategies at national level as well as at a global scale.

1.1 Renewable Energy

Renewable energy sources are indigenous, and can therefore contribute to reduce dependency on oil imports, increasing security of supply and environmental benefit. Due to these reasons, the investment towards renewable energy is drastically

© The Author(s) 2015
P. Ravindra, K.R. Jegannathan, *Production of biodiesel using lipase encapsulated in κ-carrageenan*, SpringerBriefs in Bioengineering,
DOI 10.1007/978-3-319-10822-3_1

Fig. 1.1 World marketed energy consumption (IEA outlook 2007)

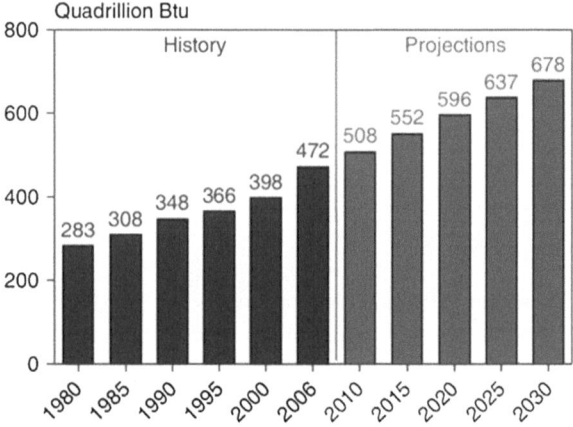

Fig. 1.2 World energy-related carbon dioxide emissions by fuel type (IEA outlook 2007)

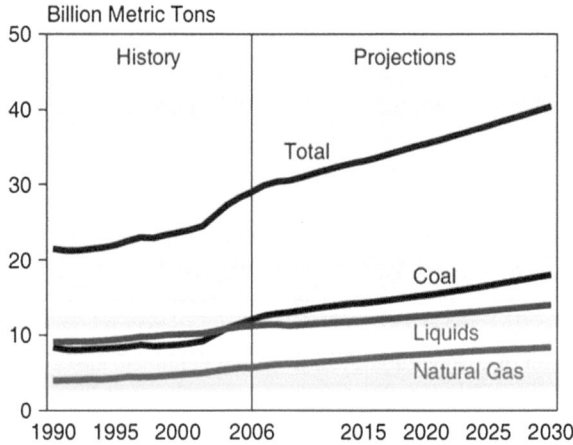

Fig. 1.3 Global investment in renewable energy (REN21 2009)

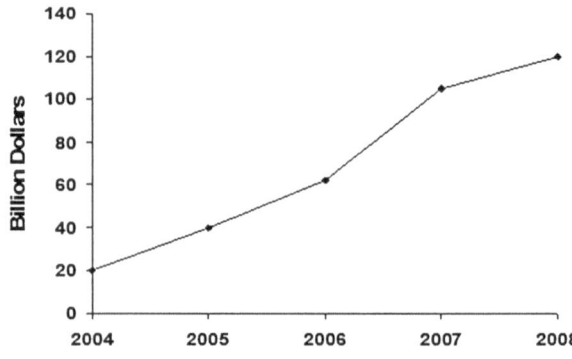

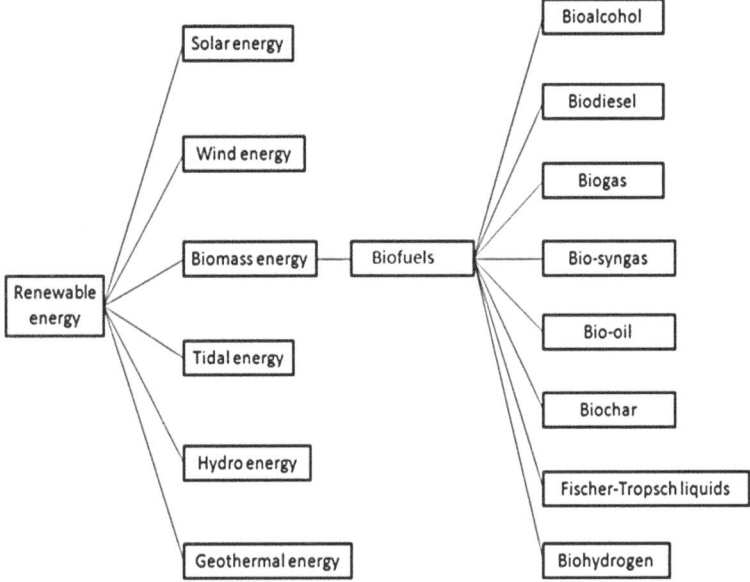

Fig. 1.4 Classification of renewable energy

increasing around the world (Fig. 1.3). Renewable energy can be classified into various types (Fig. 1.4), among which biofuels could be considered as a major energy source promoted and produced in most of the countries around the world.

1.2 Biofuels

Biofuels provide the prospect of new economic opportunities for people in rural areas, concerning job creation, greater efficiency in the general business, and protection of the environment (Demirbas 2008) (Fig. 1.5). Biofuels – liquid or gaseous fuels derived predominantly from biomass may be able to provide an alternative source of energy that could be both sustainable and without serious environmental impact. Biofuels are produced from plant oils, algal oil, animal fats, sugar beets, cereals, organic waste and the processing of biomass. The extent to which biofuels can ultimately replace fossil fuels depends on the efficiency with which they can be produced (Malcaa and Freire 2006). Biofuel research and deployment has intensified in all countries as an alternative to fossil fuel.

Global biofuel production has tripled from 4.8 billion gallons in 2000 to about 16.0 billion in 2007 with the US and Brazil contributing 75 % of world production. Biofuels include bioethanol, biodiesel, biogas, bio-synthetic gas (bio-syngas), bio-oil, bio-char, Fischer-Tropsch liquids, and biohydrogen. Among these biodiesel

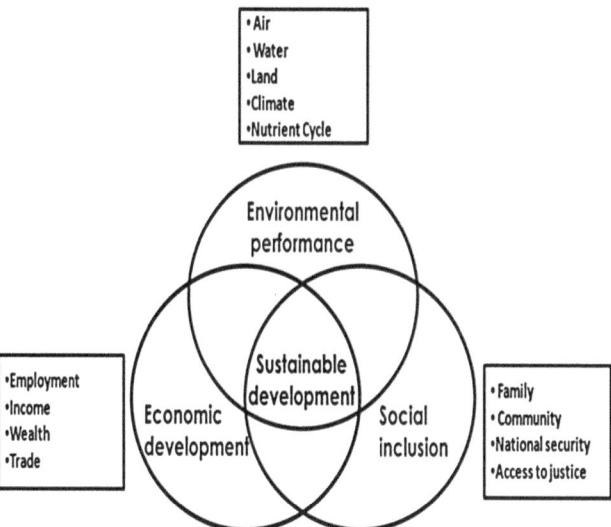

Fig. 1.5 Benefits of biofuels (Demirbas 2008)

is predominant and the biodiesel production is booming worldwide, with Europe accounting for the by far largest share of the global biodiesel production (Bacovsky et al. 2007).

1.3 History of Biodiesel

A relatively common literature statement on the early use of vegetable oils as diesel fuels is that of Rudolf Diesel, the inventor of the engine that bears his name tested "his" engine on peanut oil at the 1900 World's Fair in Paris (Knothe et al. 2005). He quotes,

> "In any case, they make it certain
> that motor-power can still be produced
> from the heat of the sun,
> which is always available for agricultural purposes,
> even when all our natural stores
> of solid and liquid fuels are exhausted."

—Diesel 1900

Initially, Rudolf Diesel was interested in running his engine on either coal or vegetable-based fuels. But, Petroleum-based fuels became the main source due to lower cost over the past century (Caye et al. 2008).

Vegetable oils were also used as emergency fuel during World War II. For example, Brazil prohibited the export of cottonseed oil in order to substitute it for imported diesel fuel. Reduced imports of liquid fuel were also reported in Argentina, necessitating the commercial exploitation of vegetable oils. China produced diesel fuel, lubricating oils from tung and other vegetable oils. However, the exigencies of the war caused hasty installation of cracking plants based on fragmentary data. Researchers in India, prompted by the events of World War II, extended their investigations on ten vegetable oils for development as a domestic fuel. Later, Work on vegetable oils as diesel fuel ceased in India when petroleum- based diesel fuel became available plentifully at low cost. The Japanese battle ship Yamato used edible refined soybean oil as bunker fuel. These events narrate the usage of vegetable oil as fuel for energy purpose in those days. However, the limitation of using vegetable oil as a fuel was its higher viscosity due to the presence of glycerol. The glycerol can be separated by a process known as transesterification (Knothe et al. 2005).

The principles of biodiesel production from vegetable oil by transesterification process have been known for a century. In 1937, The Belgian patent 422, 87 to G. Chavanne (of the University of Brussels), constitutes the first report on what is today known as biodiesel. It describes the use of ethyl esters of palm oil as diesel fuel. Even though biodiesel was patented in 1937, it was not commercially attractive due to the availability of petroleum based diesel fuel at low cost. Only after the oil crisis in 1973, research on methyl ester production technology and its application in diesel engines initiated worldwide. In Austria and France, stake holders from agriculture and industry were inspired and interest of investors arose. Pilot projects were conducted in both countries by the end of the 1980s. One of the most important results was the publication of the world´s first standard for rape oil methyl ester, which laid the basis for the approval of fatty acid methyl esters as a transport fuel and a number of international standards. Currently there are many industries producing biodiesel around the world from various oil sources (Knothe et al. 2005).

1.4   Global Biodiesel Production

Biodiesel is produced from the transesterfication of vegetable oils. Current global production of biodiesel is approximately 12 million tonnes (Fig. 1.6) and the biodiesel production capacities have increased in 2008 compared to 2007 (Fig. 1.7).

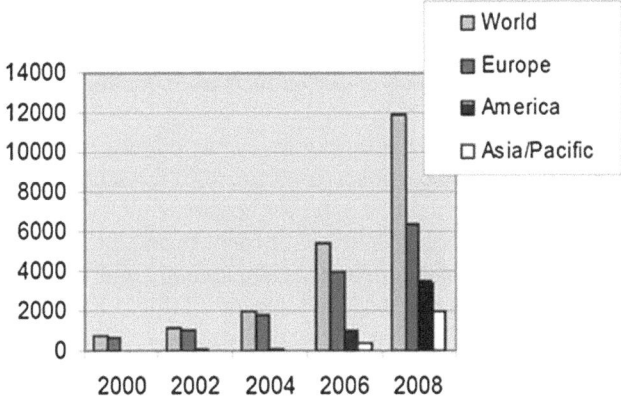

Fig. 1.6 Global biodiesel production (1,000 T) (Licht 2008)

Fig. 1.7 Global biodiesel
production capacities (10^6 T)
(Licht 2008)

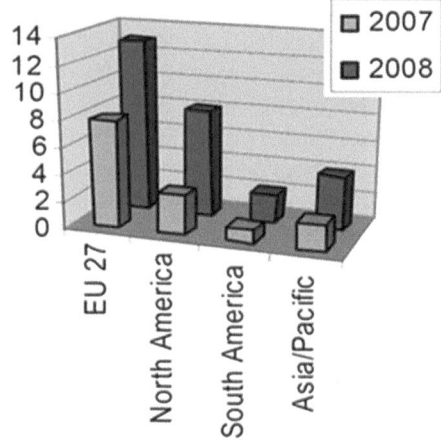

Fig. 1.8 Green house gas
emission for different fuels
(Zika et al. 2007)

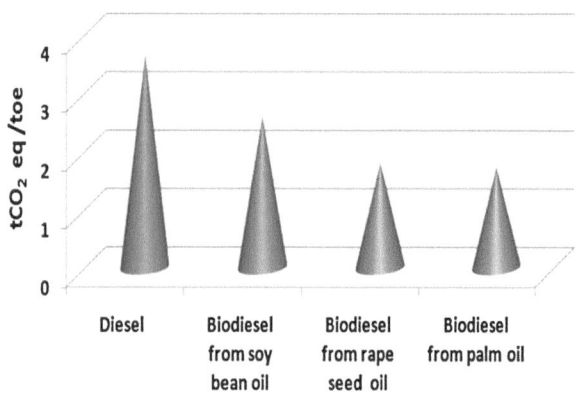

These figures are likely to increase further, due to the implementation of 20 % blend
of biofuels in conventional diesel fuel in many countries. In addition, the recent
biofuel policy 20:20:20 (20 % cut in greenhouse gas emissions for all energy compared with 1990 levels, a 20 % increase in the use of renewable energy and a 20 %
cut in energy consumption through improved energy efficiency, all by 2020) passed
by the European Union will lead to drastic increase in biodiesel production in the
world scenario.

Biodiesel can be produced by various vegetable oils and source of oil plays a
major role in biodiesel production (Al-zuhair 2007). Among the vegetable oil
sources, Palm oil has the highest oil yield per hectare of all vegetable oil feedstock.
The yield is seven times greater than that of soybean and three times that of rapeseed. In addition the biodiesel produced from palm oil emits less green house gas
compared to biodiesel from rapeseed and soybean oil (Fig. 1.8). Therefore, palm oil
would be the promising source for biodiesel production. In future, algal oil represents another source of renewable raw materials for biodiesel production. Microalgae
oil has currently received more attention as a potential feedstock owing to their high
production of lipids (Chisti 2007).

1.5 Palm Oil

1.5.1 History

The palm oil is native to West and Central Africa. Its botanical classification, *Elaeis guineensis* is derived from the Greek elaion (oil) and the specific name of guineensis is indicative of its origin from the Equatorial Guinea coast (Hartley 1988). This fruit produces two valuable vegetable oils – palm oil and palm-kernel oil. The extractable palm oil from the outer flesh (mesocarp) of the ripe orange coloured fruit constitutes approximately 20 % of the fruit's total weight and the palm kernel oil (from the nut) another 5 %. When properly cultivated, the palm oil yields up to 4.1 metric tons per hectare than any other oil-seed crop (Murphy 2009). As the palm oil has a life-span for commercial purposes of about 25 years, productivity is combined with a perennial oil source, unlike other annual oil seed crops such as soybean and rape, and is second only to soybean oil in the total world's production of vegetable oils. Over time, the palm oil has become the crop of central importance to both our daily lifestyle and too many of the great industries that man have developed (Henderson and Osborne 2000).

The demand for palm oils soon outstripped the supply available from the natural palm groves of West and Central Africa and led to the development of the palm oil as an international plantation crop. In about 1848, four trees were received by the Buitenzorg Botanical Gardens in Java. These four trees provided seed for all the palm oil grown in the Far East, where they flourished as well, if not better, than in their native Africa (Raymond 1963). Commercial development was undertaken by a Belgian firm in 1911, and large plantations were organized in Sumatra. Seed from the Sumatran plantations was the source for the large-scale planting of palm oil in Malaya (Malaysia) in 1917 in the state of Selangor.

1.5.2 Palm Oil-Global Scenario

World production of oils and fats stood at 160 million tonnes (2008). Among them, palm oil and palm kernel oil jointly accounted for 48 million tonnes (30 %), leading other oils. Soybean oil was next with 37.16 million tonnes (23 %) (Fig. 1.9). Malaysia contributed close to 11 % to the global oils and fats output through 17.7 million tonnes of palm oil. It also held 45 % of the market share, thereby maintaining dominance of the palm oil trade. Malaysian palm oil exports grew by 12.09 % over the comparative period. China, the European Union (EU), Pakistan, United States (US) and India were the biggest buyers, accounting for 60 % or 8.3 million tonnes. China remained the single largest importer, absorbing 3.79 million tonnes or 24.62 % exports. EU and Pakistan showed an intake of 2.05 million tonnes and 1.25 million tonnes respectively.

The US imported 1.04 million tonnes of Malaysian palm oil, up by 31.8 % from year 2007. This was due partly to implementation of mandatory labelling of

Fig. 1.9 World oils and fat production (MPOC 2008)

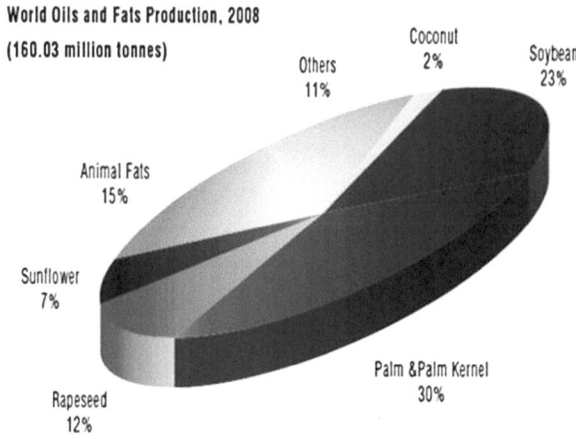

World Oils and Fats Production, 2008
(160.03 million tonnes)

Coconut 2%

Soybean 23%

Others 11%

Animal Fats 15%

Sunflower 7%

Rapeseed 12%

Palm &Palm Kernel 30%

Table 1.1 Palm oil planted area and output in Malaysia (MPOC 2008)

	Jan–Dec 2007	Jan–Dec 2008	Change	Change (%)
Planted area (ha)	4,304,914	4,487,957	183,043	4.25
Production (tonnes)				
Crude palm oil	15,823,746	17,734,439	1,910,693	12.07
Crude palm kernel oil	1,907,613	2,131,399	223,786	11.73
Closing stocks (tonnes)				
Palm oil	1,682,587	1,994,681	312,094	18.54
Palm kernel oil	268,842	348,747	79,905	29.72

the trans-fatty acid content in manufactured foods, enforced from January 2007. Higher demand was also generated by use of palm oil as feedstock for bio-fuel production (MPOC 2008).

1.5.3 Malaysian Scenario

In Malaysia, total palm oil planted area stood at 4.49 million ha, up by 4.25 % compared to the previous year. Crude palm oil (CPO) production touched 17.73 million tonnes, significantly more by 1.91 million tonnes. This was attributed to recovery in overall yield and the larger mature area. Crude palm kernel oil production rose by 11.73 % to 2.13 million tonnes from 1.91 million tonnes in 2007 (Table 1.1) (MPOC 2008). Besides producing oils and fats, at present there is a continuous increasing interest concerning palm oil renewable energy (Sumathi et al. 2008). Malaysia, with its large and growing palm oil industry (Fig. 1.10), has the potential to play a major role in the world biodiesel market.

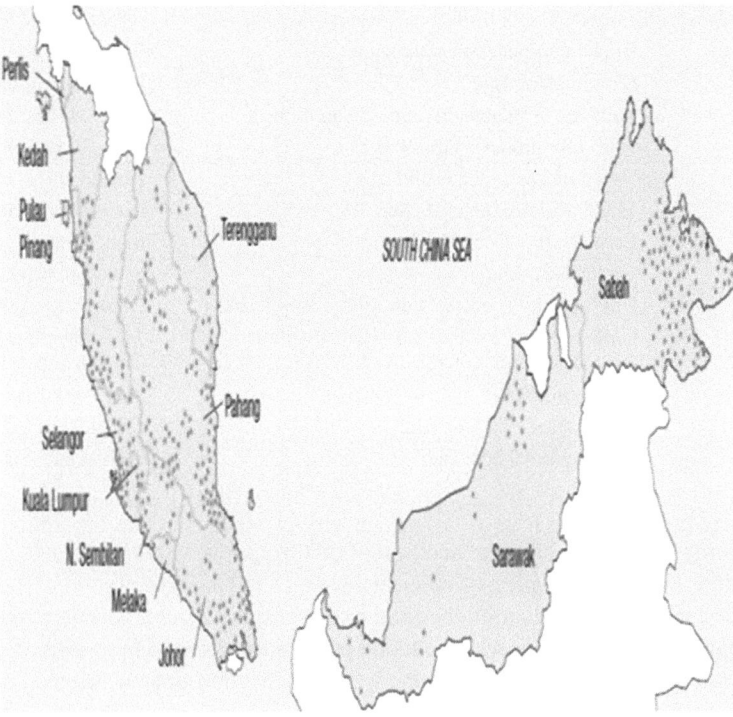

Fig. 1.10 Graphical representation of the palm oil processing plants (MPOC 2008)

1.6 Biodiesel in Malaysia

In Malaysia, there are 12 palm biodiesel operation plants (Table 1.2) and the biodiesel export from Malaysia stood at 182,108 tonnes in 2008 compared to 95,013 tonnes in 2007 respectively.

Overseas and domestic markets will remain attractive in the years to come given the EU's vote in favour of sourcing 20 % of its energy needs from renewable feedstock by 2020 (MPOC 2008) and the announcement of 5 % biodiesel blend by Malaysian government. On the other hand, production of biodiesel from palm oil would create competition of using palm oil for food. However, there should be a balance between the use of palm oil for food and fuel to maintain the demand leading to economy to the producers. Hence, switching some of the palm oil from food supply to biodiesel production will benefit the country for palm oil business by creating a demand so that the price of palm oil can be controlled profitably. Thus, biodiesel production from palm oil in Malaysia has high potential and benefits in agriculture, rural, business, employment and environment. In fact the seventh (1996–2001), eighth (2001–2005) and ninth (2005–2009) Malaysian plan emphasis

Table 1.2 Biodiesel production plants in Malaysia (Malaysia biofuels annual report 2009)

S. No	Biodiesel production plant name	Place
1	Carotino Sdn. Bhd	Pasir Gudang, Johor
2	Malaysia Vegetable oil refinery Sdn. Bhd	Pasir Gudang, Johor
3	PGEO Bioproducts Sdn. Bhd	Pasir Gudang, Johor
4	Vance Bioenergy Sdn. Bhd	Pasir Gudang, Johor
5	Mission Biotechnologies Sdn. Bhd	Petaling Jaya, Selangor
6	Carotech Bio-fuels Sdn. Bhd	Ipoh, Perak
7	Lereno Sdn. Bhd	Setiawan, Perak
8	Golden Hope Biodiesel Sdn. Bhd- Carey Island	Pulau Carey, Selangor
9	Golden Hope Biodiesel Sdn. Bhd- Panglima Island Sdn. Bhd	Teluk Panglima Garang, Selangor
10	Zoop Sdn. Bhd	Shah Alam, Selangor
11	Global Biodiesel Sdn. Bhd	Lahad Datu, Sabah
12	SPC Biodiesel Sdn. Bhd	Lahad Datu, Sabah

on energy efficiency and on generation of oils from renewable sources in an effort to reduce the rapid depletion of other fuel sources (UNDP 2007).

The current technology uses chemical catalyst for biodiesel production. The use of chemical catalyst in biodiesel production process may lead to huge pollution problems due to the soap formation in the transesterification process. Hence, development of sustainable technology is essential to achieve cleaner environment. Towards this goal, this work aims to use green technology instead of chemical technology to achieve sustainability and environmental renaissance in biodiesel sector.

1.7 White Biotechnology

White biotechnology, also known as Industrial biotechnology, is the modern use and application of biotechnology for the sustainable production of biochemicals, biomaterials and biofuels from renewable resources, using living cells and/or their enzymes. Whereas, red biotechnology is the application of biotechnology in medicine and green biotechnology is the application of biotechnology in agriculture. White biotechnology results generally in cleaner processes than chemical processes with minimum waste generation and energy use. White biotechnology results generally in cleaner processes with minimum waste generation and energy use. White biotechnology is mainly based on fermentation technology and biocatalysts. In a contained environment, genetically modified or non-GM micro-organisms (e.g. yeast, fungi and bacteria) or cell lines from animal or human origin are cultivated in closed bioreactors to produce a variety of goods. Likewise enzymes, which are derived from these (micro- organisms, are applied to catalyse a conversion in order to generate the desired products (McKinsey 2006).

The generally perceived advantage of this technology is due to the intrinsic properties of enzymes that distinguish them from conventional catalysts: First of all they

Fig. 1.11 Chemical industry impact by biotechnology (McKinsey 2006)

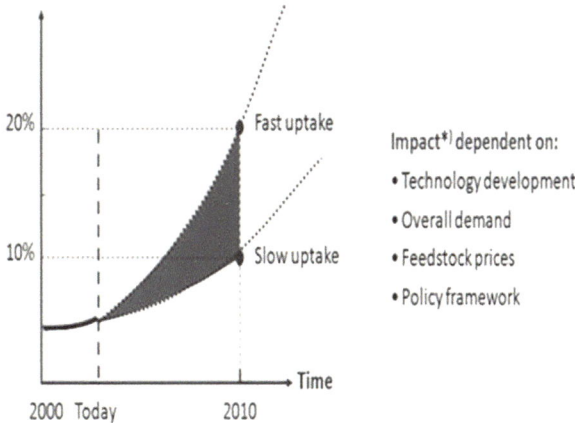

*) Impact means the use of biotechnological process steps such as fermentation, biocatalysis, etc.

usually show a high selectivity, yielding products with high contents of desired active material. Secondly, they act at comparably mild reaction conditions, such as temperatures around or slightly above room temperature, more or less neutral pH values, etc. These features can lead to simple production processes, yielding products of superior quality, without the need for multi-step synthesis or harsh reaction conditions (Thum and Oxenbøll 2008).

An estimate by McKinsey & Company shows that white biotechnology could be applied in the production of 10–20 % of all chemicals sold by the year 2010 (Fig. 1.11). The study predicts that this will be motivated by both cost reduction as well as the promise of additional revenues via new products and value added processes (McKinsey 2006). Over the past decades, enzymatic processes have gained ground from chemical processes in manufacturing in a variety of industrial branches including biodiesel. In biodiesel production chemical catalyst can be replaced by enzyme catalyst.

1.8   Biodiesel Production Using Lipase Enzymes

The first report on the application of lipase to produce methyl esters (biodiesel) dates back to 1986, British Patent GB 2 188 057 A by Choo and Ong (1986). As compared to other catalyst types, biocatalysts have several advantages. They enable conversion under milder reaction conditions. Transesterification using lipase does not lead to side reaction, forming soap. Hence, neither the ester product nor the glycerol phase has to be purified from residues or soaps unlike chemical catalyst. Therefore phase separation is easier, high-quality glycerol can be sold as a by-product, and environmental problems due to alkaline wastewater are eliminated (Wu et al. 1999). Moreover, both the transesterification of triglycerides and the esterification of free fatty acids occur in one process step. As a consequence,

Table 1.3 Comparison of the different technologies to produce biodiesel (Marchetti et al. 2008)

Variable	Alkali catalysis	Lipase catalysis
Reaction temperature (°C)	60–70	30–40
Free fatty acids in raw materials	Soaponified products	Methyl esters
Water in raw material	Interference with reaction	No influence
Yield of methyl esters	Normal	Higher
Recovery of glycerol	Difficult	Easy
Purification of methyl esters	Repeated washing	None
Production cost of catalyst	Cheap	Relatively expensive
Catalyst requirement	Low	High
Product yield	High	Low

highly acidic fatty materials, such as palm oil or waste oils, can be used without pre-treatment (Fukuda et al. 2001). In addition, many lipases show considerable activity in catalyzing transesterification with long or branched chain alcohols, which can hardly be converted to fatty acid esters in the presence of conventional alkaline catalysts (Bacovsky et al. 2007). The advantages of using a biocatalyst over chemical catalyst are listed in the Table 1.3.

However, lipase-catalyzed transesterification also entail a series of drawbacks. As compared to conventional alkaline catalysis, reaction efficiency tends to be poor, so that biocatalysts usually necessitate far longer reaction times and higher catalyst concentrations. In addition, the main hurdle to the application of lipases in industrial biodiesel production is their high price, especially if they are used in the homogenous enzyme preparations, which cannot be recovered from the reaction products. One strategy to overcome these limitations is the immobilization of lipases on a carrier, enabling the removal of the enzymes from the reaction mixture and their reuse for subsequent transesterifications (Akoh et al. 2007; Al-zuhair 2007; Jegannathan et al. 2008).

1.9 Immobilization

Immobilization refers to the localization or confinement of an enzyme on to a solid support or on a carrier matrix. The first attempt to immobilize a biocatalyst backs to 1953, while in 1969 an immobilized enzyme was used for the first time in an industrial process. Since then this technique has gained more and more importance, and now a wide variety of immobilized enzymes are employed in the food, pharmaceutical and chemical industries (Ramachandra et al. 2002). This interest is due in part to the fact that the use of lipases has the potential to be more cost effective when enzymes are employed in immobilized form rather than in free form. In principle immobilized lipase technology would facilitate the development of continuous, large-scale commercial processes which have a high efficiency per unit volume of reactor corresponding high rate of return of capital costs (Malcata and Hill 1991).

Furthermore, the use of immobilized lipases leads to a decrease in potential for contamination of the product via residual lipases, thus avoiding the need for downstream thermal treatment. It also enhances opportunities for better control of both the process and product quality (Fjerbaek et al. 2009; Akoh et al. 2007; Al-zuhair 2007; Jegannathan et al. 2008). Hence, immobilized lipase processes offer great potential for future development. Immobilized lipases prepared employing various supports and matrices have been tested for biodiesel production. However, in the current industrial development, where sustainability is given more priority, traditional carrier materials (such as anion exchange resins or polyethylene) can be replaced by renewable, readily available substances like biopolymer (Uitz 2006; Jegannathan et al. 2008).

1.10   Biopolymer Material

Biopolymers are known for their film-forming properties, which have been intensively investigated for food and non-food applications. It has been shown that a wide range of film properties can be obtained owing to the diversity of available polysaccharides (Nisperos-Carriedo 1994). Carrageenan is a generic name for a family of gel forming and viscous polysaccharides, which are obtained by extraction from certain species of the red seaweeds (Rhodophyta). They are produced on a commercial scale in Argentina, Chile, the Philippines, Indonesia, Malaysia, Morocco, France, Canada, and the North Atlantic region (Velde and Ruiter 2002).

Carrageenans are used in a wide variety of applications, especially in food products, such as frozen desserts, chocolate-milk, cottage cheese, whipped cream, yoghurt, jellies, and sauces. In addition to this, carrageenans are used in pharmaceutical and cosmetic formulations and in other industrial applications, such as in oil-well drilling fluids (Velde and Ruiter 2002). The use of carrageenan for food applications started almost 600 years ago. Due to this long and safe use, carrageenan is generally recognized as safe by experts of the US Food and Drug Administration. Since the 19th century, carrageenan has been used for industrial applications. In the 1970s, the use of carrageenan for the immobilization of enzymes and microorganisms was introduced by the pioneering work of Chibata and coworkers (Takata et al. 1977).

1.11   Research Background

Transesterification of triglycerides with alcohol in the presence of chemical catalyst or biocatalyst leads to the formation of alkyl ester commercially known as the biodiesel (Fig. 1.12) (Fjerbaek et al. 2009; Akoh et al. 2007; Al-zuhair 2007; Jegannathan et al. 2008). Production of biodiesel using alkaline catalyst has been commercially implemented due to its high conversion and low production time. For the product

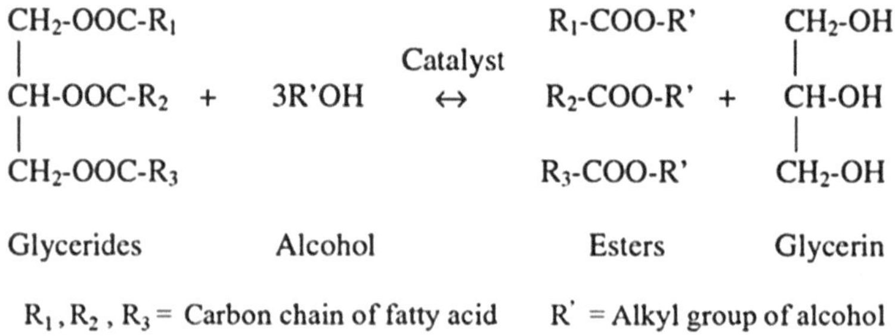

CH$_2$-OOC-R$_1$ R$_1$-COO-R'   CH$_2$-OH
| Catalyst |
CH-OOC-R$_2$ +   3R'OH   ↔   R$_2$-COO-R' + CH-OH
| |
CH$_2$-OOC-R$_3$ R$_3$-COO-R'   CH$_2$-OH

Glycerides   Alcohol   Esters   Glycerin

R$_1$, R$_2$, R$_3$ = Carbon chain of fatty acid   R' = Alkyl group of alcohol

Fig. 1.12 General scheme of transesterification reaction

and process development of biodiesel, enzymatic transesterification using lipase looks attractive and encouraging for reasons of easy product separation, minimal wastewater treatment needs, easy glycerol recovery and the absence of side reactions, unlike the chemical catalyst (Ravindra 2006; Marchetti et al. 2008).

Practical use of lipase in pseudo homogenous reaction systems presents several technical difficulties such as contamination of the product with residual enzymatic activity, and economic cost (Al-Zuhair 2007). In order to overcome this problem, the enzyme is usually used in immobilized form, so that it can be reused several times to reduce the cost, and also to improve the quality of the product by avoiding contamination. Immobilization refers to the localization or confinement of an enzyme on to a solid support or on a carrier matrix. Immobilized lipase prepared from different immobilization methods have been employed for biodiesel production. Among the immobilization methods, adsorptions on various carrier particles have been chosen by most of the researchers (Fjerbaek et al. 2009; Jegannathan et al. 2008). Other immobilization methods employed were cross-linking (Kumari et al. 2007), entrapment (Hsu et al. 2001; Noureddini et al. 2005) and encapsulation (Orcaire et al. 2006).

Encapsulation is the confinement of enzyme within a porous membrane forming a bilayer. Encapsulation can be carried out by various processes, such as coacervation phase separation, interfacial polymerization, solvent evaporation, spray coating, multiorifice centrifugation and air suspension (Benita 1996). Method of producing microcapsules is the subject of several review articles (Benita 1996; Sparks 1981; Thies 1994; Goodwin and Somerville 1974). Although, numerous methods are described in these articles, the majority are not suitable for producing large (>50 μm diameter) mononuclear microcapsules which show true shell–core morphology and are capable of containing an aqueous-based solution as a core. Such capsules can be prepared by co-extrusion (Toreki et al. 2004). The process of co-extrusion involves ejecting two liquid streams through concentric nozzles under a force. In this manner, the centre nozzle carries liquid solution to be encapsulated while the outer nozzle carries the polymer. The main advantage of this immobilization lies in the specific particle structure, in which contact between the substrate and the biocatalyst can be achieved in an appropriate way, since the biocatalyst is in solution within the core of the capsule (Jankowski et al. 1997).

Using natural polymers as a matrix for encapsulation, has several advantages like low cost, process repeatability, lack of toxicity and environmental friendly. Lipase encapsulated in κ-carrageenan has not been explored for biodiesel production elsewhere. In the present study, lipase was encapsulated in κ-carrageenan and used in the transesterification reaction of palm oil to produce biodiesel in an immobilized bioreactor. The kinetics, modelling, life cycle analysis and the economic assessment of biodiesel produced using κ-carrageenan encapsulated lipase were also studied.

1.12   Life Cycle Assessment (LCA)

As fossil fuel supplies dwindle, we will have to both reduce our consumption and look for alternative feedstock as sources of fuels and materials. In many cases, the production of bio based materials can require lower consumption of fossil fuels and other finite resources, and generate lower overall environmental impacts than alternatives. However, this should not be assumed – just because a product is made from renewable materials does not give you an ecofriendly label. Renewable materials need to be examined on a case-by-case basis (Dommett 2008).

Life cycle assessment is a technique for assessing the environmental aspects associated with a product over its life cycle. The most important applications are analysis of the contribution of the life cycle stages to the overall environmental load, usually with the aim to prioritize improvements on products or processes and comparison between products for. Every product has a life cycle stretching from the extraction or production of raw materials to final disposal. Between these stages there will be manufacturing, transport, storage and use of the product. Each of these steps will require materials and energy inputs, and may produce potentially harmful outputs to air, water and land. Life Cycle Assessment (LCA) is a method for categorizing and quantifying these inputs and outputs from 'cradle to grave' to evaluate a product's net environmental impact.

LCA is defined as the "compilation and evaluation of the inputs, outputs and potential environmental impacts of a product system throughout its life cycle". Thus, LCA is a tool for the analysis of the environmental burden of products at all stages in their life cycle – from the extraction of resources, through the production of materials, product parts and the product itself, and the use of the product to the management after it is discarded, either by reuse, recycling or final disposal. The total system of unit processes involved in the life cycle of a product is called the "product system" (Hand book on LCA 2004).

The environmental burden covers all types of impacts upon the environment, including extraction of different types of resources, emission of hazardous substances and different types of land use. It uses a holistic approach called 'cradle to grave'. One fundamental reason for choosing such an approach is related to the fact that the final consumption of products happens to be the driving force of the economy. Therefore, this final consumption offers core opportunities for indirect environmental management along the whole chain or network of unit processes related to a

Fig. 1.13 Product life cycle
model (Bhander et al. 2003)

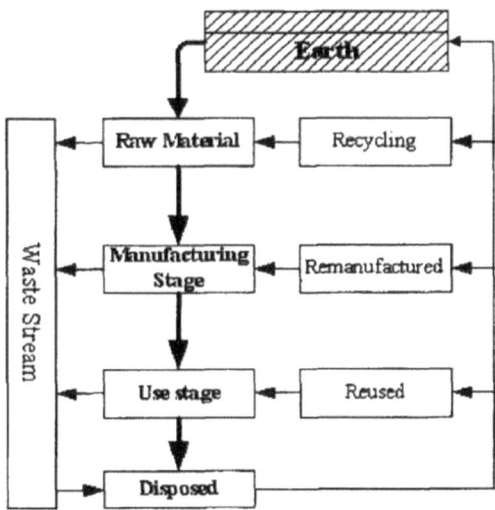

product (Hand book on LCA 2004). LCA can play a useful role in public and private
environmental management in relation to products related to an environmental
comparison between existing products and the development of new products,
eco-labelling and eco-design.

LCA study can be branched into four stages: (1) Define the goal and scope of the
study, (2) Inventory analysis, (3) Impact assessment (4) Interpretation. The first step
in LCA study is defining the goal and scope of the study. Before the study begins,
its precise purpose and intended audience should be defined. The system boundaries
of that particular system have to be mentioned clearly. The functional unit then has
to be defined, which means specifying the precise function of a product and the
quantity of product that fulfills that function. Process flow chart or the process life
cycle model (Fig. 1.13) for each system should be drawn and all the unit process,
input, output and waste disposal should be clearly mentioned. The inventory analysis
phase of an LCA study consists of collecting the data on the inputs and outputs
associated with the system under consideration available in databases and literature.
The final part of the inventory analysis involves allocating the inputs and outputs
between the main product and any co-products or by-products. The impact assessment phase of a LCA study involves evaluating the environmental significance of
the raw data you have collected (Hand book on LCA 2004).

The next step in assessing impact is characterization the conversion of inputs
or outputs into the same units of measurement. The results for each category are
converted into a convenient unit of measurement. The final part of a LCA is the
interpretation phase, which involves examining the results from the previous phases
with a critical eye to check that the conclusions you have drawn are adequately
supported by the data, and are consistent with the original goal and scope.

There are several profit and non-profit LCA software available in the market.
Each has their unique method of life cycle assessment, but the basic approach is
same for all. A list of LCA software is given in the Table 1.4.

Table 1.4 List of LCA softwares

Name of the LCA soft ware	Developers
ECO-it	PRé Consultants
EDIP	Danish EPA
EIOLCA	Carnegie Mellon University
GaBi	PE International
IDEMAT	Delft University
KCL-ECO 3.0	KCL Laboratory
LCAiT	Chalmers Industriteknik
SimaPro 7	PRé Consultants
TEAM	Ecobalance, Inc.
Umberto	Institut für Umweltinformatik
JEMAI	Research Centre for Life Cycle Assessment

1.13 Economic Assessment

Economic assessment is a systematic approach to determine the optimum use of scarce resources involving comparison of two or more alternatives, in achieving a specific objective under the given assumptions and constraints. It takes into account the opportunity costs of resources employed and attempts to measure in monetary terms the private and social costs and benefits of a project to the community or economy (Sakai et al. 2009).

Economic assessment is a key driving force supporting the development of inexpensive feedstock and process technology. Using economical assessment we can predict the cost of the process plant along with the product manufacturing cost. The economic assessment can also be used to compare the cost of product produced by different process and conditions. Although total costs of production depend heavily upon feedstock costs, there are some other considerations that must be taken into account. The main economic criteria which have to be noted are the total capital investment cost (TCC), total manufacturing cost (TMC) and total production cost (TPC) (Tsutomu et al. 2009).

1.13.1 Factors of Economic Assessment

The factors which effects the economic assessment includes, total capital investment cost, total manufacturing cost and total production cost. Capital investment cost is the cost going to be invested on a particular project for producing a product. It involves all the following cost details; equipment, installation, piping, insulation, painting, civil structure, electrical instrumentation, computer system, engineering and supervising.

Before estimating all the above mentioned cost, the capacity of the plant along with process flow chart and time frame of the reaction for batch or continuous process has to be defined. Once these parameters are defined, the capital investment cost for that defined capacity can be calculated. Basics for capital investment cost includes development of process blocks flow sheets, development of process time charts for achieving a capacity defined, development of material and energy balances for achieving a capacity defined, development of equipment lists, estimation of equipment costs, estimation of the plant costs, estimation of variable costs and estimation of fixed cost. Once the capital investment cost has been estimated, the total manufacturing cost of the product involves the following cost; raw material, utilities, man power, depreciation, repair, byproduct, interest and Tax.

Product cost : The total product cost = Total manufacturing cost − By product cost

The above mentioned cost is the product cost of a product at the factory. The market price of the product is normally higher than the factory price owing the profit margin. The profit margin is fixed based on the demand and sales of the product. An economical assessment can be done to a product using a single process or using many processes available and comparing them on the basis of feasibility among those processes. This is the main advantage of economical assessment tool, by which the cost of the product and the cheapest process can be determined (Sakai et al. 2009; Tsutomu et al. 2009).

1.14 Research Problem

The chemical production of biodiesel is a well-developed and commercialized technique that uses a low-cost catalyst and has a shorter reaction time than the enzymatic and immobilized-whole cell processes. However, chemical production also suffers from some serious disadvantages. The process operating costs are high for a number of reasons (Mittelbach and Remschmidt 2006). Various side reactions are formed which lead to soap formation, requires a separation unit to remove the precipitate formed. The use of chemical catalysts also requires additional waste water treatment which is a burden to production and also to the environment. The byproduct glycerol produced during transesterification is impure and needs further purification and a higher quantity of alcohol above the stoichiometric is required to obtain higher conversion (Ma and Hanna 1999; Fukuda et al. 2001; Barnwal and Sharma 2005).

The enzymatic processing of biodiesel addresses many of the problems associated with chemical processing. It requires only moderate operating conditions and yields a high-quality product with a high level of conversion and the life cycle assessment of enzymatic biodiesel production has more favourable environmental consequences in abiotic depletion, global warming, ozone layer depletion, human toxicity, fresh water aquatic ecotoxicity, photochemical oxidation, acidification and eutrophication (Harding et al. 2008). The chemical processing problems of waste water treatment are lessened and soap formation is not an issue, meaning that waste oil with higher FFA can be used as the feedstock. The byproduct glycerol does not require any purification and it can be sold at higher price.

However, soluble enzymatic processing is not perfect. It is costly, the enzyme cannot be recycled and its removal from the product is difficult. For these reasons, immobilized enzymatic process has been developed which retains the advantages of the soluble enzymatic process and reuse of the enzyme is possible which decreases the enzyme cost, the biodiesel produced does not contain any enzyme residue and the activity of the enzyme can be increased by immobilization. The drawbacks of the immobilized enzyme process are mass transfer limitation, enzyme leakage, the lack of a versatile commercial immobilized enzyme and some of immobilization methods involve toxic chemicals.

1.15 Approach

To overcome the drawbacks of the immobilized enzyme in biodiesel production process, an attempt is made to use a degradable biopolymer (κ-carrageenan) as a carrier for lipase immobilization in biodiesel production and to encapsulate lipase in κ-carrageenan by coextrusion technique to achieve immobilization at milder conditions and safer disposal of catalyst

1.16 Scope

The scope of this research was to develop a novel technique for lipase immobilization by encapsulation, to study the physical properties and stability characteristics of the encapsulated lipase, to produce and optimize process parameters such as effect of oil: methanol ratio, effect of water content, effect of temperature, effect of enzyme loading, effect of mixing intensity, effect of reaction time and effect of flow rate of biodiesel from palm oil using encapsulated lipase in a stirred tank batch immobilized reactor and in recirculated packed bed immobilized reactor, to determine the kinetic constants and reaction time for stirred tank batch reactor and comparison of predicted data with experimental data, to study the diffusion effects of encapsulated lipase in biodiesel production, to study the life cycle assessment of biodiesel production and to study the economic assessment of biodiesel production.

References

Akoh CC, Chang SS, Lee GG, Shaw JJ (2007) Enzymatic approach to biodiesel production. J Agri Food Chem 55:8995–9005
Al-zuhair S (2007) Production of biodiesel: possibilities and challenges. Biofuels Bioprod Biorefin 1:57–66
Bacovsky D, Körbitz W, Mittelbach M, Wörgetter M (2007). Biodiesel production: technologies and European providers. IEA Task 39 Report T39-B6

Barnwal BK, Sharma MP (2005) Prospects of biodiesel production from vegetable oils in India. Renew Sust Energy Rev 9:363–378

Benita S (1996) Microencapsulation methods and industrial applications. Marcel Dekker, New York

Bhander GS, Hauschild M, McAloone T (2003) Implementing Life Cycle Assessment in Product Development. Environ Prog 22:255–267

Caye MD, Nghiem PN, Terry HW (2008) Biofuels engineering process technology. McGraw-Hill, New York

Chisti Y (2007) Biodiesel from microalgae. Biotechnol Adv 25:294–306

Choo YM, Ong SH (1986) Transesterification of fats and oils. British Patent GB 2 188 057 A

Demirbas A (2008) Biofuels sources, biofuel policy, biofuel economy and global biofuel projections. Energy Convers Manage 49:2106–2116

Dommett L (2008) An introduction to Life Cycle Assessment. Biofuels Bioprod Biorefin 2:385–388

Fjerbaek L, Christensen KV, Norddahl B (2009) A review of the current state of biodiesel production using enzymatic transesterification. Biotechnol Bioeng 102:1298–1315

Fukuda H, Kondo A, Noda H (2001) Biodiesel fuel production by transesterification of oils. J Biosci Bioeng 92:405–416

Goodwin JT, Somerville GR (1974) Microencapsulation by physical methods. Chem Mag 623–626

Hand book on Life Cycle Assessment (2004) Eco-Efficiency in industry and science. Kluwer Academic, New York

Harding KG, Dennis JS, Blottnitz HV, Harrison STL (2008) A life-cycle comparison between inorganic and biological catalysis for the production of biodiesel. J Clean Prod 16:1368–1378

Hartley CWS (1988) The oil palm. Longman, San Francisco

Henderson J, Osborne DJ (2000) The palm oil in all our lives: how this came about. Endeavour 24:63–68

Hsu A, Jones K, Marmer WN, Foglia TA (2001) Production of alkyl esters from tallow and grease using lipase immobilized in a phyllosilicate sol-gel. J Am Oil Chem Soc 78:585–588

IEA (2007) Energy technology essentials: biomass for power generation and CHP. International Energy Agency Report

Jankowski T, Zielinska M, Wysakowska A (1997) Encapsulation of lactic acid bacteria with alginate/starch capsules. Biotechnol Techniq 1:31–34

Jegannathan KR, Abang S, Poncelet D, Chan ES, Ravindra P (2008) Production of biodiesel using immobilized lipase- a critical review. Crit Rev Biotechnol 28:253–264

Knothe G, Gerpen JV, Krahl J (2005) The biodiesel hand book. American Oil Chemical Society Press, Champaign

Kumari V, Shah S, Gupta MN (2007) Preparation of biodiesel by lipase-catalyzed transesterification of high free fatty acid containing oil from Madhuca indica. Energy Fuel 21:368–372

Licht FO (2008) World ethanol & biofuels. Report, no. 16

Ma F, Hanna A (1999) Biodiesel production: a review. Bioresour Technol 70:1–15

Malaysia biofuels annual report. 2009. GAIN, Kuala Lumpur

Malcaa J, Freire F (2006) Renewability and life-cycle energy efficiency of bioethanol and bio-ethyl tertiary butyl ether (bioETBE): assessing the implications of allocation. Energy 31:3362–3380

Malcata FX, Hill CG (1991) Use of a lipase immobilized in a membrane reactor to hydrolyze the glycerides of butter oil. Biotechnol Bioeng 38:853–868

Marchetti JM, Miguel UV, Errazu AF (2008) Techno-economic study of different alternatives for biodiesel production. Fuel Proces Technol 89:740–748

McKinsey (2006) White biotechnology: gateway to a more sustainable future. EuropaBio, Brussels

Mittelbach M, Remschmidt C (2006) Biodiesel: the comprehensive handbook. Martin Mittelbach, Graz

MPOC (2008) Malaysian palm oil council Annual Report. MPOC, Kuala Lumpur

Murphy DJ (2009) Global oils yields: have we got it seriously wrong? Inform 20:499–500

Nisperos-Carriedo M (1994) Edible coatings and films based on polysaccharides. Edible coatings and films to improve food quality. Lancaster, Technomic

Noureddini H, Gao X, Philkana RS (2005) Immobilized pseudomonas cepacia lipase for biodiesel fuel production from soybean oil. Bioresour Technol 96:769–777

Orcaire O, Buisson P, Pierre AC (2006) Application of silica aerogel encapsulated lipases in the synthesis of biodiesel by transesterification reactions. J Mol Catal B: Enzym 42:106–113

Ramachandra MV, Jayadev B, Muniswaran PKA (2002) Hydrolysis of oils by using immobilized lipase enzyme: a review. Biotechnol Bioprocess Eng 7:57–66

Ravindra P (2006) Biofuels scenario in Asian countries. Proceedings of 2006 World Congress on Industrial Biotechnology and Bioprocessing. Toronto, Canada

Raymond WD (1963) The palm oil industry. Trop Sci 3:69–89

REN21 (2009) Renewables Global Status Report: Update.

Sakai T, Kawashima A, Koshikawa T (2009) Economic assessment of batch biodiesel production processes using homogeneous and heterogeneous alkali catalysts. Bioresour Technol 100: 3268–3276

Sheehan J, Cambreco V, Duffield J, Garboski M, Shapouri H (1998) An overview of biodiesel and petroleum diesel life cycles. A report by US Department of Agriculture and Energy 1–35

Sparks RE (1981) Microencapsulation in encyclopedia of chemical technology. John Wiley & Sons, New York

Srivastava A, Prasad R (2000) Triglycerides-based diesel fuels. Renew Sust Energy Rev 4:111–113

Sumathi S, Chai SP, Mohamed AR (2008) Utilization of palm oil as a source of renewable energy in Malaysia. Renew Sust Energy Rev 12:2404–2421

Takata I, Tosa T, Chibata I (1977) Screening of matrix suitable for immobilization of microbial cells. J Solid Phase Biochem 2:225–236

Thies C (1994) Microencapsulation: mini answers to major problems. Today's chemist 40

Thum O, Oxenbøll KM (2008) Biocatalysis – a sustainable method for the production of Emollient Esters. Int J Appl Sci 134:44–47

Toreki W, Manukian A, Strohschein R (2004) Hydrocapsules and method of preparation thereof. US Patent 6,780,507

Tsutomu S, Ayato K, Tetsuya K (2009) Economic assessment of batch biodiesel production processes using homogeneous and heterogeneous alkali catalysts. Bioresour Technol 100:3268–3276

Ture S, Uzan D, Ture IE (1997) The potential use of sweet sorghum as a non-polluting source of energy. Energy 22:17–19

Utz R (2008) Ph.D. Dissertation. Karl-Franzens-University

UNDP (2007) Malaysia generating renewable energy from palm oil wastes. United Nations Development Programme (UNDP) report, Malaysia

Velde FV, Ruiter GAD (2002) Polysaccharides II: polysaccharides from eukaryotes. Wiley-VCH, Weinheim

Wu WH, Foglia TA, Marmer WN, Phillips JG (1999) Optimizing production of ethyl esters of grease using 95 % ethanol by response surface methodology. J Am Oil Chem Soc 76:517–521

Zika E, Papatryfo I, Wolf O, Manuel GB, Alexander JS, Bock AK (2007) Consequences, opportunities, and challenges of modern biotechnology of Europe. JRC-European commission report

Chapter 2
Literature Review

Abstract The literature review of biodiesel production is presented in this chapter. In the first part, the various catalysts which are being used for biodiesel production was reviewed in detail. In the second part the need for immobilized enzyme, the various immobilization techniques and immobilized enzyme used for biodiesel production were reviewed critically. The third part in the literature review was devoted to κ-carrageenan, the enzymes, the methods used for immobilization using κ-carrageenan and applications were reviewed. In the fourth part the factors effecting the biodiesel production using immobilized lipase was reviewed critically and various suggestions were given based on the literature. The latter parts were devoted to the immobilized bioreactors, enzyme kinetics, life cycle assessment, and economics assessment.

The origin of all fuel and biofuel compounds is ultimately the sun, as solar energy. It is captured and stored as organic compounds through photosynthetic processes. Certain biofuels, such as oils produced by plants and algae, are direct products of photosynthesis. These oils can be used directly as fuel or transesterified to biodiesel. Other biofuels like ethanol and methane are produced as organic substrates. They are fermented by microbes under anaerobic conditions. Hydrogen gas can be produced by both routes, such as, by photosynthetic algae and cyanobacteria under certain nutrient or oxygen-depleted conditions, by bacteria and archae utilizing organic substrates under anaerobic conditions (Caye et al. 2008) (Fig. 2.1).

Recent incentives to reduce greenhouse gases, particularly carbon dioxide, have led to great interest in vegetable-based fuels because of a plant's inherent ability to capture solar energy through photosynthetic pigments (via light reactions) while efficiently sequestering carbon dioxide from the atmosphere as their primary carbon source (via dark reactions). This carbon is then biologically converted to high-energy starches, celluloses, proteins, and oils as storage and structural compounds (Tillman et al. 2006) (Fig. 2.2).

Biofules are produced from vegetable-based raw materials and considered as environmental friendly substitute for fossil fuel. Biofuels include bioethanol, biodiesel, biogas, bio-synthetic gas (bio-syngas), bio-oil, bio-char, Fischer-Tropsch liquids, and biohydrogen. A comparison of biofuel energy contents reveal that for liquid fuels, such as biodiesel, gasoline, and diesel have energy densities in the

© The Author(s) 2015

23

P. Ravindra, K.R. Jegannathan, *Production of biodiesel using lipase encapsulated in κ-carrageenan*, SpringerBriefs in Bioengineering, DOI 10.1007/978-3-319-10822-3_2

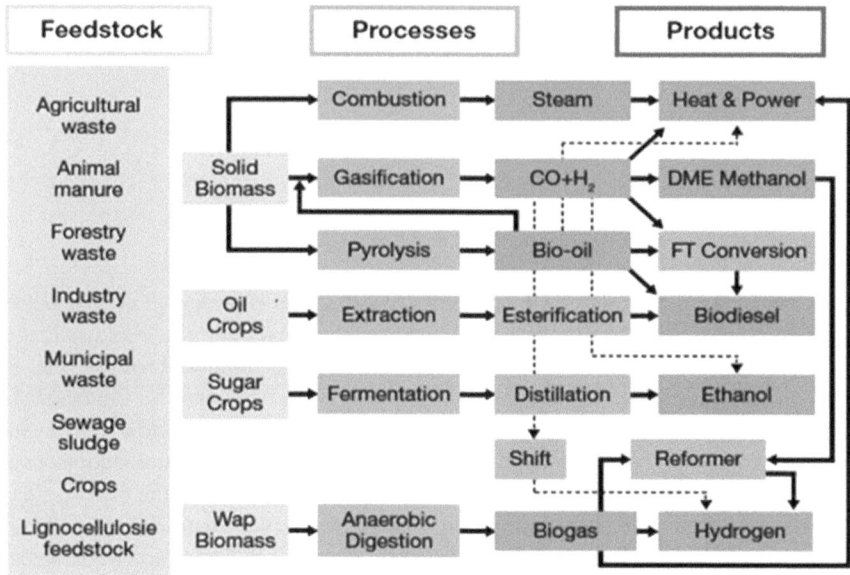

Fig. 2.1 Overview of biomass conversion path and biofuels production process (International Energy Agency 2007)

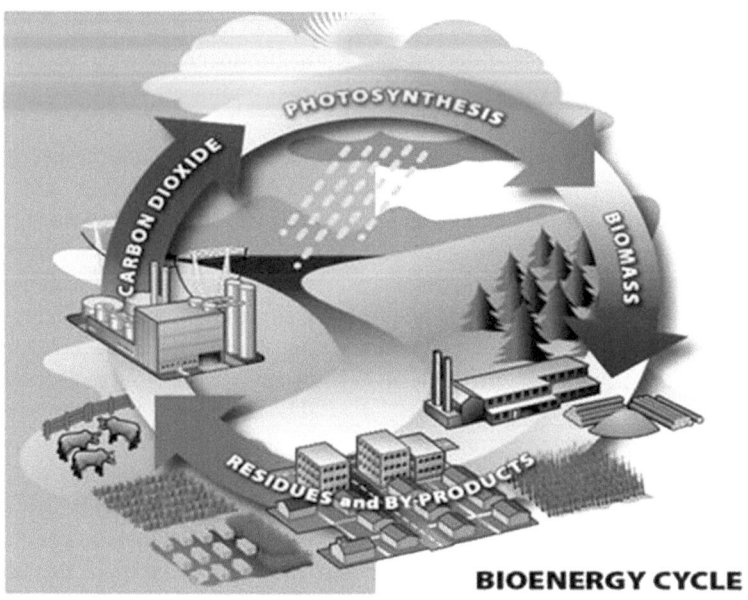

Fig. 2.2 Bioenergy cycle (Tillman et al. 2006)

Table 2.1 Energy density values for common fuels (At standard temperature and pressure) (Caye et al. 2008)

Fuel source	Energy density (kJ/g)
Hydrogen	143.0
Methane (natural gas)	54.0
Diesel	46.0
Gasoline	44.0
Soybean biodiesel	40.2
Ethanol	129.6
Methanol	22.3

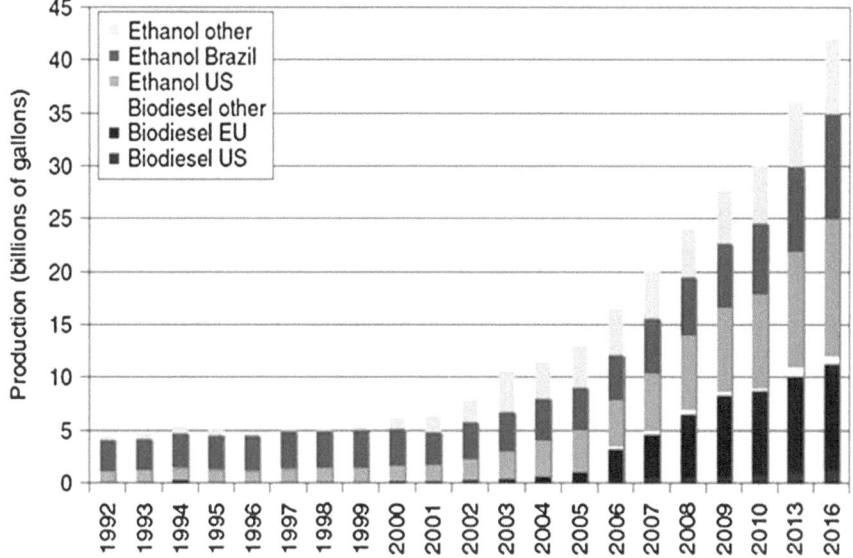

Fig. 2.3 World biodiesel and ethanol historical production and projections (Licht 2008)

40–46 kJ/g range, expressed on a mass basis. Hydrogen gas has the highest energy density of common fuels (Table 2.1). Biodiesel fuel contains 13 % lower energy density than petroleum diesel fuel, but combusts more completely and has greater lubricity (Caye et al. 2008).

Biofuel production, if approached in a sustainable manner, can be more environmentally benign than fossil fuel technologies (Tillman et al. 2006). Among biofuels, the production of bioethanol and biodiesel have increased over the past decade (Fig. 2.3) and expected to increase in the future due to the implementation of biofuel blend policy (Table 2.2).

Among biodiesel and bioethanol, the production of bioethanol suffers from product inhibition; ethanol in concentrations above a certain threshold value in the reactor will drastically reduce the fermentative capacity of the organisms used. In addition, the storage of ethanol is costly due to its hygroscopic and corrosive nature. However, intensive research is being conducted in microbial strain development towards

Table 2.2 Biofuel blending policies in various countries (REN21 2009)

Country	Policy
Australia	E2 in New South Wales, increasing to E10 by 2011; E5 in Queensland by 2010
Argentina	E5 and B5 by 2010
Bolivia	B20 by 2015
Brazil	E22 to E25 existing (slight variation over time); B3 by 2008 and B5 by 2013
Canada	E5 by 2010 and B2 by 2012; E7.5 in Saskatchewan and Manitoba; E5 by 2007 in Ontario
Chile	E5 and B5 by 2008 (voluntary)
China	E10 in 9 provinces
Colombia	E10 and B10 existing
Dominican Republic	E15 and B2 by 2015
Germany	E5.25 and B5.25 in 2009; E6.25 and B6.25 from 2010 through 2014
India	E5 by 2008 and E20 by 2018; E10 in 13 states/territories
Italy	E1 and B1
Jamaica	E10 by 2009
Korea	B3 by 2012
Malaysia	B5 by 2008
Paraguay	B1 by 2007, B3 by 2008, and B5 by 2009; E18 (or higher) existing
Peru	B2 in 2009; B5 by 2011; E7.8 by 2010
Philippines	B1 and E5 by 2008; B2 and E10 by 2011
South Africa	E8–E10 and B2–B5 (proposed)
Thailand	E10 by 2007 and B10 by 2012; 3 % biodiesel share by 2011
United Kingdom	E2.5/B2.5 by 2008; E5/B5 by 2010
United States	Nationally, 130 billion litres/year by 2022 (36 billion gallons); E10 in Iowa, Hawaii, Missouri, and Montana; E20 in Minnesota; B5 in New Mexico; E2 and B2 in Louisiana and Washington State; Pennsylvania 3.4 billion litres/year biofuels by 2017 (0.9 billion gallons)
Uruguay	E5 by 2014; B2 from 2008–11 and B5 by 2012

efficient production of bioethanol by increasing the ethanol resistance of the microbial stain. However, in case of biodiesel these drawbacks are eliminated. Biodiesel seems to be the most likely technology which is capable of scaling up large-scale production in a controlled and cost-effective manner (Fjerbaek et al. 2009; Akoh et al. 2007; Al-zuhair 2007; Jegannathan et al. 2008). In addition glycerol, the byproduct of biodiesel production can be converted to ethanol by anaerobic fermentation (Yazdani and Gonzalez 2007) would favour in the reduction of production cost. It also has the advantage of safer handling and storage and distribution along with other benefits.

The benefits of biodiesel include:

• Reduced vehicle emissions
• Reduced engine wear because of the fuel's excellent lubricity (ability to lubricate the engine and fuel system)

- Increased safety in storage and transport because the fuel is nontoxic and biodegradable
- Increased value for farm products
- Reduced dependence on foreign oil suppliers and associated price fluctuations

2.1   Biodiesel

Biodiesel, a hot topic in every country's policy agenda is a renewable and environment friendly substitute for petroleum based diesel fuel (Jegannathan et al. 2008). It is nearly a colourless liquid made from the transesterification of vegetable oils and animal fats and has properties similar to petroleum-based diesel. In particular, it has a relatively high cetane number and about 90 % of the energy content of petroleum diesel, making it an attractive direct substitute or blend component (Concawe 2006). Chemically, biodiesel is equivalent to fatty acid methyl esters (FAME) or ethyl esters (FAEE), produced out of triacylglycerols via transesterification or out of fatty acids via esterification. In Fig. 2.4 the formula scheme for the production of fatty acid methyl esters (FAME) out of triacylglycerols is shown. Fatty acid methyl esters today are the most commonly used biodiesel species, whereas fatty acid ethyl esters (FAEE) so far have been only produced in laboratory or pilot scale.

2.2   Process Description

Presently, the industrial production of biodiesel is a chemical process based on the transesterification of various oils using alkaline or acid catalysts. However, recent laboratory-scale research has aimed to develop production techniques with different

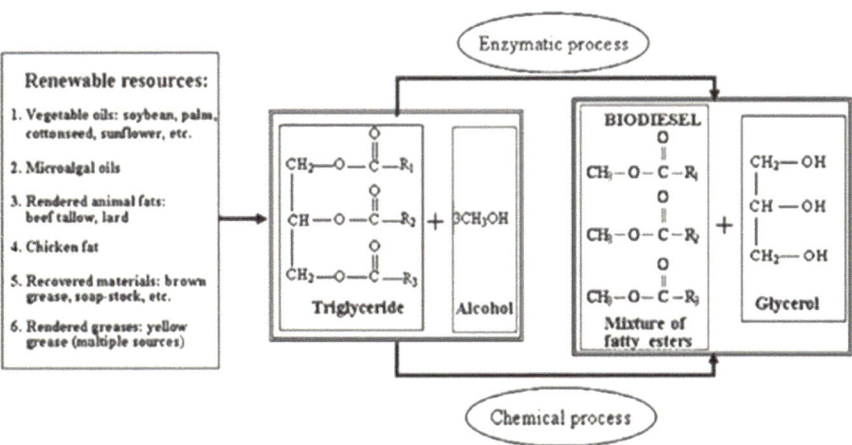

Fig. 2.4 Overall scheme of biodiesel by transesterfication

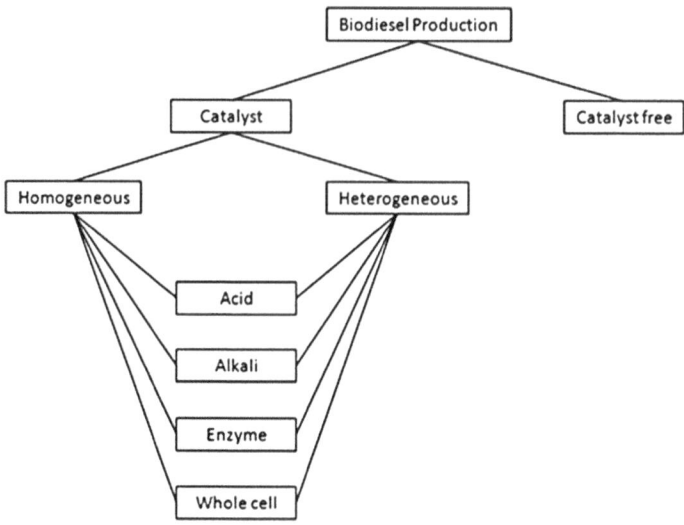

Fig. 2.5 Classification of catalyst used for biodiesel production

type of catalysts. The various types of catalyst used for biodiesel production are alkali catalyst, acid catalyst, catalyst free, enzyme catalyst and whole cell enzyme catalyst. Various catalyst used for biodiesel production can be classified into three types namely; homogenous catalyst, heterogeneous catalyst and catalyst free (Fig. 2.5). Each process has its own advantages and disadvantages. Every catalytic process differs in their process parameters. The scope of this thesis is limited to enzymatic process and hence all the other catalyst process are not discussed in detail, however an over view of the catalyst used and their impact on biodiesel production are discussed in the following sections.

2.2.1 Homogeneous Alkaline Catalyst

Alkaline or basic catalysis is by far the most commonly used reaction type for biodiesel production. The main advantage of this form of catalysis is the high conversion under mild conditions in comparatively short reaction time (Freedman et al. 1986). Moreover, alkaline catalysts are less corrosive to industrial equipment, and thus enable the use of less expensive carbon-steel reactor material. The main drawback of the catalyst is the sensitivity of alkaline catalysts to free fatty acids contained in the feedstock material which leads to increased soap formation (Mittelbach and Remschmidt 2006; Fjerbaek et al. 2009; Akoh et al. 2007; Al-zuhair 2007; Jegannathan et al. 2008). Various alkaline catalysts have been employed for biodiesel production. A list of catalysts used and their impact on biodiesel production is summarized in (Tables 2.3 and 2.4)

Table 2.3   Different type of catalyst used for biodiesel production (Caye et al. 2008)

Type of catalyst		Name of catalyst
Homogeneous	Alkali	Sodium hydroxide
		Potassium hydroxide
		Sodium methoxide
		Potassium methoxide
	Acid	Conc. sulphuric acid
		p-Toluene-sulphonic acid
	Organic	Lipase enzyme
		Whole cell
Heterogeneous	Alkali	Egg shell
		Alkali metal carbonates and hydrogen Carbonates (Na_2CO_3, $NaHCO_3$, K_2CO_3, $KHCO_3$)
		Alkali metal oxides (K_2O)
		Alkali metal salts of carboxylic acids (Cs-laurate)
		Alkaline earth metal alcoholates
		Alkaline earth metal carbonates ($CaCO_3$)
		Alkaline earth metal oxides (CaO, SrO, BaO)
		Alkaline earth metal hydroxides $Ba(OH)_2$
		Alkaline earth metal salts of carboxylic Acids (Ca- and Ba- acetate)
		Strong anion exchange resins Amberlyst (A 26, A 27)
		Zink oxides/ aluminates
		Metal phosphates (ortho-phosphates of aluminium, gallium or iron (III))
		Transition metal oxides, hydroxides and Carbonates (Fe_2O_3 ($+Al_2O_3$), Fe_2O_3, Fe_3O_4, FeOOH, NiO, Ni_2O_3, $NiCO_3$, $Ni(OH)_2$ Al_2O_3)
		Silicates and layered clay minerals (Na /K silicate Zn-, Ti- or Sn- silicates and aluminates)
		Zeolite catalysts (Titanium-based zeolites, faujasites)
		Shrimp Shell catalysts
Heterogeneous	Acid	Acidic ion exchange resins
		Transition metal salts of amino acids (Zn- and Cd-arginate)
		Transition metal salts of fatty acids (Zn- and Mn-palmitates and stearates)
		Sulfonated zirconia
		Sulfonated tin oxide
		Amberlyst-15
		Naphion NR50
	Organic	Sugar catalyst (D-glucose)
		Immobilized lipase enzyme
		Immobilized whole cell

Table 2.4 Comparison of catalyst type used in biodiesel production (Jegannathan et al. 2009)

Parameter	Catalyst type		Level	Remarks
Catalyst cost	Homogenous	Acid	Low	Market price compared to organic catalyst
		Alkali	Low	Market price compared to organic catalyst
		Organic	High	Market price compared to acid and alkali catalyst
	Heterogeneous	Acid	low	Price reduces due to reuse
		Alkali	low	Price reduces due to reuse
		Organic	Medium	Price reduces due to reuse
	Catalyst free		Nil	No catalyst used
Equipment cost	Homogenous	Acid	Very High	corrosion demands costly equipments
		Alkali	Very High	corrosion demands costly equipments
		Organic	Low	No corrosion
	Heterogeneous	Acid	Medium	Less corrosion
		Alkali	Medium	Less corrosion
		Organic	Low	No corrosion
	Catalyst free		Very High	Demands costly equipments and high safety systems
Operating cost	Homogenous	Acid	High	High energy demands due to high reaction temperature
		Alkali	High	High energy demands due to high reaction temperature
		Organic	Low	Low energy demands due to low reaction temperature
	Heterogeneous	Acid	Very High	High energy demands due to high reaction temperature
		Alkali	Very High	High energy demands due to high reaction temperature
		Organic	Low	Low energy demands due to low reaction temperature
	Catalyst free		Very high	High energy demands due to high reaction temperature and pressure
Product purity	Homogenous	Acid	Low	Due to side reactions
		Alkali	Low	Due to side reactions
		Organic	Low	No side reactions
	Heterogeneous	Acid	High	No side reactions
		Alkali	High	No side reactions
		Organic	High	No side reactions
	Catalyst free		Very High	No side reactions

(continued)

Table 2.4 (continued)

Parameter	Catalyst type		Level	Remarks
Waste water treatment cost	Homogenous	Acid	High	Acid use
		Alkali	High	Alkali use
		Organic	Low	Less chemicals used
	Heterogeneous	Acid	High	Acid use
		Alkali	High	Acid use
		Organic	Low	Less chemicals used
	Catalyst free		Nil	No chemicals used
Environmental benefits	Homogenous	Acid	Low	High waste disposal
		Alkali	Low	High waste disposal
		Organic	High	Low waste disposal
	Heterogeneous	Acid	Low	High waste disposal
		Alkali	Low	High waste disposal
		Organic	High	Low waste disposal
	Catalyst free		Very High	High solvent use
Production inhibition	Homogenous	Acid	Medium	Due to side reactions
		Alkali	Medium	Due to side reactions
		Organic	Low	No side reactions
Production inhibition	Heterogeneous	Acid	Low	No side reactions
		Alkali	Low	No side reactions
		Organic	Low	No side reactions
	Catalyst free		Nil	No side reactions
Continuous process	Homogenous	Acid	Not possible	Cannot be reused
		Alkali	Not possible	Cannot be reused
		Organic	Not possible	Can be reused
	Heterogeneous	Acid	Possible	Can be reused
		Alkali	Possible	Can be reused
		Organic	Possible	Can be reused
	Catalyst free		possible	Solvents can be recovered and reused

2.2.2 Homogeneous Acid Catalyst

Acid-catalyzed transesterification is usually far slower than alkali catalyzed reactions and requires higher temperatures and pressures as well as higher amounts of alcohol. The typical reaction conditions for homogeneous acid-catalyzed methanolysis are temperatures up to 100 °C and pressures up to 5 bars in order to keep the alcohol as liquid (Mittelbach et al. 1983). Another disadvantage of acid catalysis is the increased formation of unwanted secondary products, such as dialkyl ethers or glycerol ethers.

2.2.3   Homogeneous Enzyme Catalyst

Use of lipase enzyme from various microorganisms has become a topic in biodiesel production (Bacovsky et al. 2007). Lipases are enzymes which catalyze both the hydrolytic cleavage and the synthesis of ester bonds in glycerol esters. As compared to other catalyst types, biocatalysts have several advantages. They enable conversion under mild temperature, pressure- and pH-conditions. Neither the ester product nor the glycerol phase has to be purified. It does not lead to side reaction forming unwanted secondary products. Therefore phase separation is easier, high-quality glycerol can be obtained as a by-product, and environmental problems due to alkaline and acid wastewater are eliminated (Wu et al. 1999; Mittelbach and Remschmidt 2006; Fjerbaek et al. 2009; Akoh et al. 2007; Al-zuhair 2007; Jegannathan et al. 2008). The main hurdle in application of lipases for industrial biodiesel production is their high price, especially if they are used in the soluble form, which cannot be recovered from the reaction products.

2.2.4   Homogeneous Whole Cell Microorganisms

Biodiesel production using whole cell microorganisms has been reported in the literature. Instead of using a soluble lipase enzyme, the lipase producing microorganism *Rhizopus oryzae* cells have been inoculated in the reaction medium containing oil and alcohol. Biodiesel conversion similar to other catalyst has been reported (Sriappareddy et al. 2007).

Apart from the above mentioned disadvantages of homogenous catalysts, the major disadvantage is the fact that homogenous catalysts cannot be reused. Moreover, catalyst residues have to be removed from the ester product, usually necessitating several washing steps, which increases production costs. Thus there have been various attempts at simplifying product purification by applying heterogeneous catalysts, which can be recovered by decantation or filtration or alternatively used in a fixed-bed catalyst reactor. These advantages have made the researchers to work on heterogeneous catalyst (Sriappareddy et al. 2007; Sriappareddy et al. 2008).

2.2.5   Transesterification Without Catalysts

Transesterification of triglycerides with lower alcohols also proceeds in the absence of a catalyst, provided reaction temperature and pressures are high enough. Ester conversion up to 85 % after ten hours of reaction has been reported for non-catalytic methanolysis of soybean oil at 235 °C and 62 bars (Diasakou et al. 1998). The advantages of not using a catalyst for transesterification are that high-purity esters and soap-free glycerol are produced. Especially in the recent years reactions using supercritical methanol without any catalyst have been reported, however, the reaction conditions are very extreme (Kusdiana and Saka 2001). The high excess of methanol which has to be used during supercritical transesterification seems to make the process not economically feasible.

2.2.6 Heterogeneous Alkali Catalyst

The alkaline heterogeneous catalysts used are listed in the Table 2.3. Alkali metal- and alkaline earth metal carbonates and oxides used were most cited. However, the high reaction temperatures and pressures and the high alcohol volumes required in this technology are likely to prevent its commercial application. On the other hand, the use of strong alkaline ion-exchange resins is limited by their low stability at temperatures higher than 40 °C (Bondioli 2004).

2.2.7 Heterogeneous Acid Catalyst

Various Heterogeneous acid catalysts had been investigated for biodiesel production (Table 2.3). The advantage of acid heterogeneous catalyst include efficient conversion of waste cooking and rendered oils high in free fatty acids to biodiesel with simultaneous esterification and transesterification reactions and the relative ease recovery and regeneration of catalyst. The disadvantage with the heterogeneous acid catalysts is the loss of activity after each use due to inhibitors that poison the catalyst with highly absorbed residues, and potential desorption of the acid active groups (López et al. 2007).

2.2.8 Heterogeneous Whole Cell Micro Organism

Similar to enzyme catalyst the whole cell micro organisms cannot be reused due to their smaller size. If the micro organisms are not removed it would contaminate the product. Thus, immobilization of lipase producing organism was carried out. In a study reported by Sriappareddy et al. (2008) *Rhizopus oryzae* cells were immobilized in polyurethane biomass particle using glutaraldehyde solution to catalyze methanolysis and the process yielded methyl ester content in the range 70–80 % at 72 h. Though, use of lipase producing organism seems to be advantageous the materials used for immobilization are toxic which may lead to unsafe disposal problems.

2.2.9 Heterogeneous Enzyme Catalyst

The high cost of soluble lipase enzyme has made the researcher to look for heterogeneous lipase catalyst. This heterogeneous catalyst would allow the catalyst to be reused several times favouring the production cost. Heterogeneous enzyme catalyst can be prepared by immobilizing lipase in a suitable carrier. Several works have been reported for biodiesel production using immobilized lipase on various carrier matrices. Production of biodiesel using immobilized lipase is the subject of the review article (Jegannathan et al. 2008; Fjerbaek et al. 2009; Akoh et al. 2007; Al-zuhair 2007). This thesis deals with the production of biodiesel using an immobilized lipase; hence a detailed review on this topic is presented in the later session.

2.3   Immobilization

Immobilization refers to the localization or confinement of an enzyme on to a solid support or on a carrier matrix. The choice of a carrier is dependent upon several factors, namely: mechanical strength, microbial resistance, thermal stability, chemical durability, chemical functionality hydrophobic/ hydrophilic character, ease of regeneration, loading capacity, and cost, which is important in industrial processing applications (Karube et al. 1977). Enzyme immobilization is experiencing an important transition. Combinations of approaches are increasingly applied in the design of immobilized enzyme by rational combination of basic immobilization techniques i.e., noncovalent adsorption, covalent binding, entrapment, and encapsulation. The availability of a robust immobilized enzyme at an early stage definitely enables early insight into process development, and saves cost for process development and production (Cao et al. 2003). The following sections provides a review on the various types of immobilization techniques used for enzymatic production of biodiesel, the achievements and drawbacks, as well as the various factors, which affect biodiesel production by using an immobilized enzyme.

2.3.1   Various Lipase Immobilization Techniques Used for Biodiesel Production

Immobilized enzymes are defined as "enzymes physically confined or localized in a certain defined region of space with retention of their catalytic activities, and which can be used repeatedly and continuously." The term 'immobilized enzyme' was recommended at the First Enzyme Engineering Conference in 1971. In general, the methods for enzyme immobilization can be classified into two basic categories, based on chemical retention and physical retention (Bommarius and Riebel-Bommarius 2000) as shown in Fig. 2.6. An immobilized enzyme has to perform two essential functions: namely, the non-catalytic functions that are designed to aid separation and the catalytic functions that are designed to convert the targeting substrates within a desired time and space (Cao 2005). The last few years have witnessed the design of high activity biocatalyst preparations for use in nonaqueous systems (Shah et al. 2004). Various immobilization techniques have been employed on lipase used for biodiesel production and they are discussed as follows.

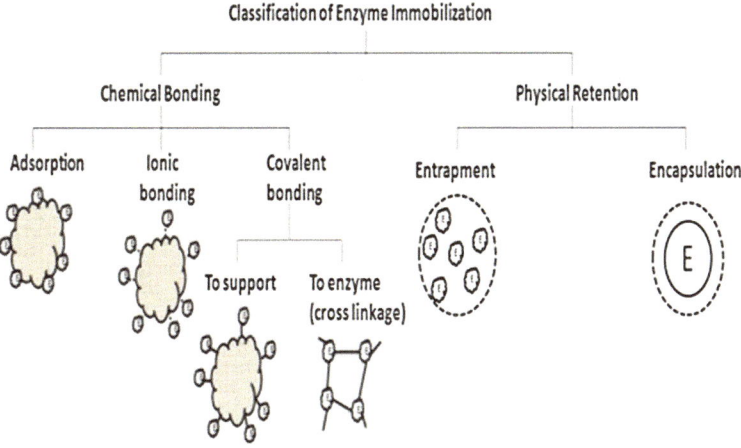

Fig. 2.6 Classification of immobilization methods (Jegannathan et al. 2008)

2.3.2 *Adsorption*

Adsorption is the attachment of enzymes on the surface of support particles by weak forces, such as van der Waals or dispersion forces. Adsorption is the most straight-forward immobilization procedure. The preparation is easy and the associated costs are small. This immobilization method involves no toxic chemical and the resulted immobilized enzyme does not experience internal mass transfer limitations, unlike cross-linking and entrapment. Various carrier particles have been explored for immobilization of lipase for biodiesel production. An extensive list of the type of carrier used has been summarized in Table 2.5. Among them are such as Toyonite 200-M, Celite, Accurel, Diatonomous earth, Polypropylene EP 100, Textile mem-brane, Hydrotalcite, Silica gel, Acrylic resin, Anion resin, Microporous polymeric matrix, Mg–Al hydrotalcite (Iso et al. 2001; Shah et al. 2004; Yang et al. 2006; Yesiloglu 2004; Salis et al. 2005; Hsu et al. 2001; Nie et al. 2006; Yagiz et al. 2007; Wang et al. 2006; Talukder et al. 2006; Halim and Kamaruddin 2008; Dizge et al. 2009; Zeng et al. 2009).

In general, the conversions of biodiesel from various vegetables and waste oils using the enzyme immobilized in this form ranges from 76 %to 100 %. The effect of polar and non polar properties of resin as a carrier on the degree of immobilization has also been studied (Yang et al. 2006). The degree of immobilization was high when lipase was adsorbed onto a non-polar resin with a pore diameter of 8.5–9.5 nm. It was reported that the pore diameter of resin influences the degree of immobilization where degree of immobilization increases with increasing pore diameter (Yang et al. 2006).

Even though adsorption has various advantages like commercial availability and high activity for biodiesel production, the enzyme could be stripped off the support

Table 2.5 Production of biodiesel using immobilized lipase enzyme by various immobilization techniques (Jegannathan et al. 2008)

IM	Carrier used	Source of enzyme	a	Oil	Acyl acceptor	Solvents	b	c	d	X	Y	e	References
A	Toyonite-200 M	*Pseudomonas Fluorescens*	9.4	Sunflower	1-propanol		1:3	60	20	91	Increases	10	Iso et al. 2001
A	Celite	*Pseudomonas Cepacia*	10	Jatropha	Ethanol		1:4	50	12	98	Increases	4	Shah and Gupta 2006
A	Macroporous anion exchange resin	*Mucor miehei*	20	Sunflower	Ethanol	Petroleum ether	1:11	45	5	82	Increases	NA	Mittelbach 1990
A	NA	*Candida Antarctica*	1.6	Cotton seed	Methanol	t-Butanol	1:4	50	24	95	NA	NA	Rayon et al. 2007
A	NA	*Candida Antarctica*	3	Rapeseed	Methanol	t-Butanol	1:4	35	12	95	Increases	16	Li et al. 2006
A	Macro porous acrylic resin	*Candida Antarctica*	10	Jatropha	Ethyl acetate		1:11	50	12	91.3	NA	12	Mukesh et al. 2007
A	Macro porous acrylic resin	*Candida Antarctica*	4	waste cooking palm oil	Methanol	t-Butanol	1:4	40	12	88	Decreases	NA	Halim and Kamaruddin 2008
A	Polypropylene EP 100	*Pseudomonas fluorescens*	10	Sunflower	Methanol	Hexane	1:4.5	40	48	91	NA	NA	Soumanou and Bornscheuer 2003
A	Acrylic resin	*Candida antarctica*	4	Palm	Methanol	THF	1:3	40	40	97	Decreases	NA	Talukder et al. 2006
A	Silica gel	*Candida antarctica*	5	Soybean oil deodorizer distillate	Methanol	t-Butanol	1:3.9	40	25	94	NA	NA	Wang et al. 2006
A	Acrylic resin	*Candida antarctica*	2	Soybean	Methanol	Ionic liquids	1:4	50	12	80	NA	NA	Sung et al. 2007
A	Celite -545	*Chromobactrium viscosum*	10	Jatropha	Ethanol		1:4	40	10	92	Increases	NA	Shah et al. 2004
A	Anion resin	*Porcine pancreatic*	10	Sunflower	Ethanol		1:3	45	7	80	NA	2	Yesiloglu 2004
A	NA	*Candida antarctica*	30	Soybean	Methyl acetate		1:12	40	14	92	NA	NA	Xu et al. 2003
A	Nonpolar resin	*Candida sp. 99-125*	25	Soybean	Methanol	Hexane	1:3	40	28	98.8	Increases	13	Yang et al. 2006

IM	Support	Enzyme	a	Oil	Alcohol	Solvent	b	c	d	X	Y	e	Reference
A	Diatomaceous earth	*Pseudomonas cepacia*	1.4	Sunflower	2-Butanol		1:3	40	6	100	Increases	NA	Salis et al. 2005
A	Acrylic resin	*Candida antarctica*	30	Soybean	Methyl Acetate		1:12	40	14	92	NA	100	Du et al. 2004
A	Acrylic resin	*Candida antarctica*	10	Crude Jatropha	Methanol	2-Propanol	1:4	50	8	92.8	NA	12	Mukesh et al. 2006
A	Textile membrane	*Candida sp. 99–125*	20	Salad	Methanol	Hexane	1:3	40	30	96	Increases	NA	Lu et al. 2007
A	Macroporous anion resin	*Candida antarctica*	5	Palm kern oil	Ethanol	Supercritical CO_2	1:10	40	4	63	NA	NA	Oliveira and Oliveira 2001
A	Hydrotalcite	*Thermomyces lanuginosus*	4	Waste cooking	Methanol		1:4	45	105	92.8	NA	4	Yagiz et al. 2007
CL	Glutaraldehyde	*Pseudomonas cepacia*	10	Madhuca	Ethanol		1:4	40	2.5	92	NA	NA	Kumari et al. 2007
ET	Hydrophobic sol–gel	*Pseudomonas cepacia*	5	Soy bean	Methanol		1:7.5	35	30	56	Increases	4	Noureddini et al. 2005
ET	Phyllosilicate sol–gel	*Pseudomonas cepacia*	57	Tallow and grease	Ethanol		1:4	50	20	94	NA	5	Hsu et al. 2001
EP	Silica aerogel	*Burkholderia cepacia*	2.4	Sunflower	Methyl acetate	Isooctane	1:3	NA	360	64	NA	NA	Orcaire et al. 2006

a: Percentage of enzyme used (w/w of oil)

b: Oil: Alcohol Molar Ratio

c: Optimum Temperature (°C)

d: Optimum Reaction Time (h)

e: Number of reuse with Residual activity >65 %

NA: Not Available

THF: Tetrahydrofuran

IM: Immobilization method

A: Adsorption

CL: Cross-linking

ET: Entrapment

EP: Encapsulation

X: Conversion (%)

Y: Effect of water on conversion

during the reaction due to the direct shear involved between the support and the impeller as the adsorption basically occurs as a result of weak forces. In such a case the loss in the activity of enzyme was due to leaching and not due to the deactivation of enzyme (Yadav and Jadhav 2005). Depending on the strength of the interaction between the enzyme and a particular support, the immobilization process can produce distortions of the protein structure. These distortions are more effective at low loadings and cause enzyme erosion (Bosley and Peilow 1997). Hence the stability of immobilized enzyme using adsorption is very low which makes the reuse limited. In addition, the size of the adsorbed enzyme is very small which would create reuse problems and unfit for industrial applications.

2.3.3 Covalent Binding

This method is based on the formation of covalent bonds between a support material and some functional groups of the amino acid residues on the surface of the enzyme. Usually, the support has to be first activated by a specific reagent, to make its functional groups strongly electrophilic; these groups are then allowed to react with strong nucleophilic groups of the enzyme. The advantage of this method is the strength of the bond and the consequent stability of immobilization; in a recent study by Dizge et al. (2009) *Thermomyces lanuginosus* lipase was covalently attached onto Micro porous polymeric matrix containing aldehyde functional group which was synthesized using styrene, divinylbenzene, and polyglutaraldehyde. The production of biodiesel using the covalent immobilized lipase showed yields of 97 % from sunflower oil and 90.2 % from waste cooking oil (Dizge et al. 2009). However, the disadvantages are the higher costs and this method involves toxic chemicals which are not environment friendly.

2.3.4 Cross-Linking

The cross-linking method is based on the formation of intermolecular cross-linkages between the enzyme molecules by means of bifunctional or multifunctional reagents such as Glutaraldehyde, bisdiazobenzidine, hexamethylene diisocyanate etc. Cross-linked enzyme aggregates are matrix free immobilized preparations. Generally, the first step of the immobilization process is to precipitate the enzyme using acetone and this produces physical aggregates of the enzyme. These aggregates are then cross-linked with Glutaraldehyde to form a more robust structure. The application of this biocatalyst design for the production of biodiesel has been explored (Kumari et al. 2007). The use of cross-linked enzyme aggregates accelerated the rate of transesterification and a conversion of 92 % has been obtained. However, one of the intrinsic drawbacks for cross linked enzyme aggregates is that their particle size is usually below 10 µm. Thus, difficulties arise when they are used in heterogeneous reaction systems, where the substrate particle and the cross linked enzyme aggregates particles might be in the same range. This can create problems in separation of immobilized enzyme from the product for the continuous use (Cao et al. 2003). In addition the chemicals used for cross linkage are toxic which may create disposal problems and hence not environmental benign.

2.3.5   Entrapment

Entrapment of lipase entails capture of the lipase within a matrix of polymer (Xavier et al. 1990). The lipase immobilized by entrapment is much more stable than physically adsorbed lipase. This method uses a relatively simple procedure and the immobilized lipase maintains its activity and stability (Kennedy et al. 1990). A novel procedure for entrapment of *Pseudomonas cepacia* lipase within a phyllosilicate sol-gel matrix with tetramethylorthosilicate as precursor has been developed (Hsu et al. 2001). Lipase from *Pseudomonas cepacia* was entrapped within a sol-gel polymer matrix, prepared by polycondensation of hydrolyzed tetramethylorthosilicate and iso-butyltimethoxysilane. The immobilized enzyme was used in transesterification of soybean oil and a conversion of around 67 % was achieved. The low conversion of ester using immobilized lipase by entrapment was due to the poor diffusion and erosion of enzyme from the surface of the support during the processing procedures (Noureddini et al. 2005). However, a disadvantage of this method is that a large pore size could cause enzyme leakage whereas a small pore size could prevent the diffusion of large substrate molecules into the matrix to reach the biocatalyst (Velde and Ruiter 2002).

2.3.6   Encapsulation

Encapsulation is the confinement of enzyme with in a porous membrane forming a bilayer. Encapsulation avoids direct contact between the enzyme and the bulk medium. It also provides a cage to avoid the enzyme from leaching out (Yadav and Jadhav 2005). Production of biodiesel using encapsulated lipase in silica aerogel has shown a conversion of 56 %. The immobilized enzyme could be recycled several times without any apparent mechanical deterioration by wear (Orcaire et al. 2006). On the other hand a stronger diffusion limitation with encapsulated lipase occurred by a high protein concentration in the enzyme which clogs the pores in the matrices. It is worthwhile to produce an encapsulated enzyme with smaller size to overcome the mass transfer problems and to use a purified enzyme to avoid clogging (Orcaire et al. 2006).

2.3.7 Other Immobilization Techniques

The immobilization of enzyme by using a combination of different immobilization technique is known as 'hybrid immobilization' (Fig. 2.7). Hybrid immobilization has given promising results on an industrial scale in fields like food (Reyed 2007) and pharmaceuticals (Posorske 1984; Bonrath et al. 2002). In this technique, two immobilization methods are combined together, for example when an immobilized enzyme prepared via adsorption is encapsulated or an immobilized enzyme prepared by adsorption is entrapped or an immobilized enzyme prepared by entrapment is encapsulated it is an hybrid immobilization (Fig. 2.7). This approach was recently explored for transesterification of p-chlorobenzyl alcohol with vinyl acetate to give p-chlorobenzyl acetate using lipase adsorbed on hexagonal mesoporous silica followed by encapsulation on calcium alginate (Yadav and Jadhav 2005). The hybrid immobilization system showed 68 % conversion and excellent reusability with a decrease of only 4 % in overall conversion after the fourth reuse. The potential of this technique could be explored for biodiesel production. For example, it could be used to solve the leakage of enzyme immobilized through adsorption by providing a porous membrane through encapsulation.

Similarly, protein coated micro crystals are becoming popular for non-aqueous systems. Protein coated micro crystals have negligible mass transfer limitations due to their smaller size and high activity compared to cross-linked enzyme aggregates (Kumari et al. 2007). The preparation of protein coated micro crystals involves the mixing of enzyme solution with a concentrated solution of a salt, sugar or amino acid. The combined aqueous mixture is then added drop wise with rapid mixing to water-miscible organic solvent like acetone or 1-Propanol (kreiner et al. 2001)

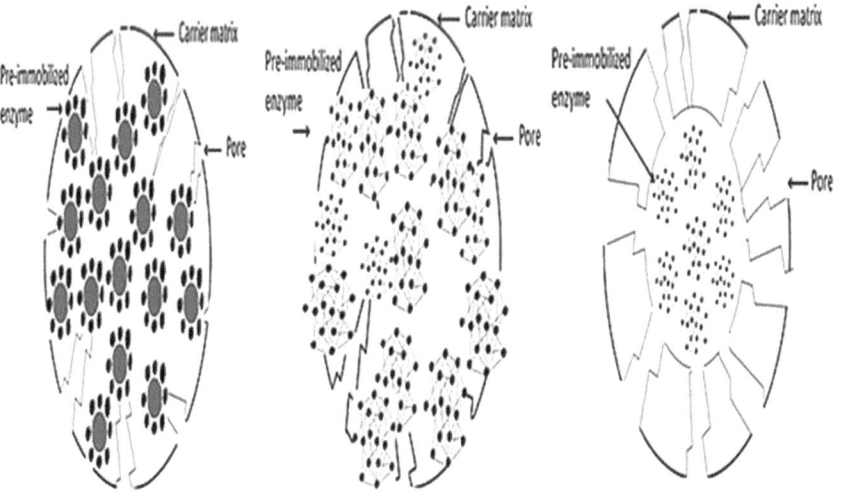

Entrapped pre-immobilized enzyme   Entrapped pre-immobilized enzyme   Encapsulated pre-immobilized enzyme

Fig. 2.7 Hybrid immobilization methods (Jegannathan et al. 2008)

2.4   Factors Affecting the Production of Biodiesel Using Immobilized Lipase

2.4.1   Pretreatment of Immobilized Lipase

Most of the commercial available lipase is in powder form. It is necessary to dissolve the lipase enzyme in a coupling media before immobilization. The type of coupling media used could influence the activity of the lipase. Both aqueous and non-aqueous coupling media have been used for dissolving the lipase enzyme. Higher ester conversion was obtained when non aqueous (heptane) coupling media was used compared to aqueous media (buffer) for immobilization of *Candida* sp. in a resin (Yang et al. 2006). The possible reason for higher conversion with heptane could be that, the treatment of lipase with polar organic solvent changes the lipase conformation from the less hydrophobic-closed form (active site is covered by lid) to more hydrophobic open form (active site is opened), favouring the binding of hydrophobic substrate to lipase (Chamorro et al. 1998; Colton et al. 1995).

On the other hand the activation of immobilized enzyme was enhanced by pretreatment of lipase in methyl oleate and soybean oil (Samukawa et al. 2000; Dong et al. 2006). The pretreatment of immobilized *Candida antarctica* lipase in isopropanol has also shown higher methyl ester conversion. In a recent study Lu et al. (2007) concluded that the pretreatment of immobilized lipase in solutions of $CaCl_2$ and $MgCl_2$ could improve the lipase activity, methanol tolerance and operational stability for biodiesel production. However, the pretreatment of lipase increases the cost of the production process.

2.4.2   Feedstock

Various vegetable oils can be used for the production of biodiesel (Table 2.5). The majority of studies reported the use of soybean oil, sunflower oil., palm oil, rape seed oil, cotton seed oil and Jatropha oil (Talukder et al. 2006; Rayon et al. 2007; Li et al. 2006; Shah and Gupta 2006; Mukesh et al. 2007) using immobilized lipase. In general, there are no technical restrictions on the use of vegetable oils for biodiesel production. However, the main constraint for biodiesel production may be the cost of the feedstock and availability. Al-Zuhair (2007) suggests considering palm oil as a favourable feed stock for biodiesel production. Palm oil has the highest yield compared to that of other vegetable oils (Table 2.6).

The high value of edible vegetable oil as a food product makes production of a cost-effective fuel very challenging. It is more reasonable to use Jatropha oil, as edible oils are not in surplus supply (Shah and Gupta 2006). Jatropha oil has an estimated annual production potential of 200 thousand metric tonnes in India (Srivastava and Prasad 2000). It can be grown in waste land with minimum amount of water and fertilizers, unlike sunflower or soybean. It grows rapidly, takes approximately

Table 2.6 List of oil producing crops and their yields

Plant	Botanical name	Yield kg Oil/hectare
Palm oil	*Elaeis guineensis*	5,000
Macauba palm	*Acrocomia aculeate*	3,775
Pequi	*Caryocar brasiliense*	3,142
Buriti palm	*Mauritia flexuosa*	2,743
Oiticia	*Licania rigida*	2,520
Coconut	*Cocos nucifera*	2,260
Avocado	*Persea Americana*	2,217
Brazil nut	*Bertholletia excelsa*	2,010
Macadamia nut	*Macadamia terniflora*	1,887
Jatropha	*Jatropha curcas*	1,590
Babassu palm	*Orbignya martiana*	1,541
Jojoba	*Simmondsia chinensis*	1,528
Pecan	*Carya illinoensis*	1,505
Bacuri	*Platonia insignis*	1,197
Castor bean	*Ricinus communis*	1,188
Gopher plant	*Euphorbia lathyris*	1,119
Piassava	*Attalea funifera*	1,112
Olive tree	*Olea europaea*	1,019
Rapeseed	*Brassica napus*	1,000
Opium poppy	*Papave somniferum*	978
Peanut	*Arachis hypogaea*	890
Cocoa	*Theobroma cacao*	863
Sunflower	*Helianthus annuus*	800
Rice	*Oriza sativa L.*	696
Buffalo gourd	*Cucurbita foetidissima*	665
Safflower	*Carthamus tinctorius*	655
Crambe	*Crambe abyssinica*	589
Sesame	*Sesamum indicum*	585
Camelina	*Camelina sativa*	490
Mustard	*Brassica alba*	481
Coriander	*Coriandrum sativum*	450
Pumpkin seed	*Cucurbita pepo*	449
Euphorbia	*Euphorbia lagascae*	440
Hazelnut	*Corylus avellana*	405
Linseed	*Linum usitatissimum*	402
Coffee	*Coffea arabica*	386
Soybean	*Glycine max*	375
Hemp	*Cannabis sativa*	305
Cotton	*Gossypium hirsutum*	273
Calendula	*Calendula officinalis*	256
Kenaf	*Hibiscus cannabinus L.*	230
Rubber seed	*Hevea brasiliensis*	217
Lupine	*Lupinus albus*	195
Palm	*Erythea salvadorensis*	189
Oat	*Avena sativa*	183
Cashew nut	*Anacardium occidentale*	148
Corn	*Zea mays*	145

2–3 years to reach maturity and it could generate economic yields. It has a productive lifespan in excess of 30 years. The fatty acid composition of Jatropha oil is similar to other edible oils but the presence of some anti-nutritional factors such as, toxic Phorbol esters renders this oil unsuitable for cooking purposes (Shah et al. 2004). Jatropha oil is thus a promising candidate for biodiesel production in terms of availability and cost.

On the other hand, there are large amount of low cost oils and fats, such as restaurant waste and animal fats that could be converted to biodiesel. The problem with processing these low-cost oils and fats is that they contain large amounts of free fatty acids that cannot be converted to biodiesel using an alkaline catalyst (Canakci and Gerpen 2001). Whereas, the oil with high free fatty acids content can be converted to esters by using immobilized lipase. The use of waste cooking oil for biodiesel production could reduce production cost and favours the environment. However, the adequate and sustainable supply of the waste oils must be ensured for large scale production.

In future, there will be an increase demand for land for the production of vegetable oils. Therefore, it is important to prioritize processes, production systems and products that are efficient with regard to the land area used and their environmental impact. Based on these criteria, algal oil represents another source of renewable raw materials for biodiesel production. Microalgae oil has currently received more attention as a potential feedstock owing to their high production of lipids (Chisti 2007). Algal oil is largely produced through substrate feeding and heterotrophic fermentation. If algal production could be scaled up industrially, less than 6 million hectares would be necessary worldwide to meet current fuel demands, amounting to less than 0.4 % of arable land (Sheehan et al. 1998).

Feed stock plays a major role in the biodiesel production. Hence, it is desirable to choose a feed stock which is locally available so that the cost of the production would decrease considerably. For example, Malaysia is rich in palm oil production, hence the availability of feed stock would be throughout the year and the price of the palm oil would be comparatively low compared to other oils. Thus palm oil would be the best candidate as a feedstock for biodiesel production in Malaysia. Similarly, in United States soybean oil would be the best choice.

2.4.3 Lipase Enzyme

The main natural function of lipases (triacylglycerols ester hydrolases EC (3.1.1.3) is to catalyze the hydrolysis of long-chain triacylglycerols (TAG). Contrary to many other enzymes, they show remarkable levels of activity and stability in non-aqueous environments, which facilitates the catalysis of several unnatural reactions such as esterification and transesterification. Literature reveals the relation between lipase structures and their catalytic ability (Cecilia et al. 2007). The overall structure of the triacylglycerol lipases can be described as a structure with a central L-sheet with the active serine placed in a loop termed the catalytic elbow. Above the serine a hydrophobic cleft are present or formed after activation of the enzyme (Svendsen 2000). The hydrophobic cleft is an elongated pocket suitable for acyl moieties to fit into. The activation, which is often necessary for the lipase enzyme is the movement of a lid. *Thermomyces lanuginose* lipase has an active site and a lid on the surface of the enzyme. *Pseudomonas* and *Candida antarctica* lipase has an active site and a funnel-like lid. *Candida rugosa* lipase has an active site at the end of a tunnel containing the lid in its external part (Pleiss et al. 1998). The structural peculiarities of lipase from different sources might be the reason for showing different activity in different substrates.

The mechanism of lipase involves the Asp-His-Ser catalytic triad acting as a charge – relay system (Bommarius and Riebel-Bommarius 2000). The carboxylate group on aspartic acid is hydrogen-bonded to histidine, and the nitrogen on histidine is hydrogen-bonded to the alcohol on serine. The first step in the reaction is to make the serine alcohol a better nucleophile. This task is performed by histidine, which completely pulls the proton off the serine alcohol, forming an oxyanion. The serine oxyanion then attacks the substrates carbonyl carbon, forming a tetrahedral intermediate 1 (Fig. 2.8). The created oxyanion is stabilized by nearby amino acids

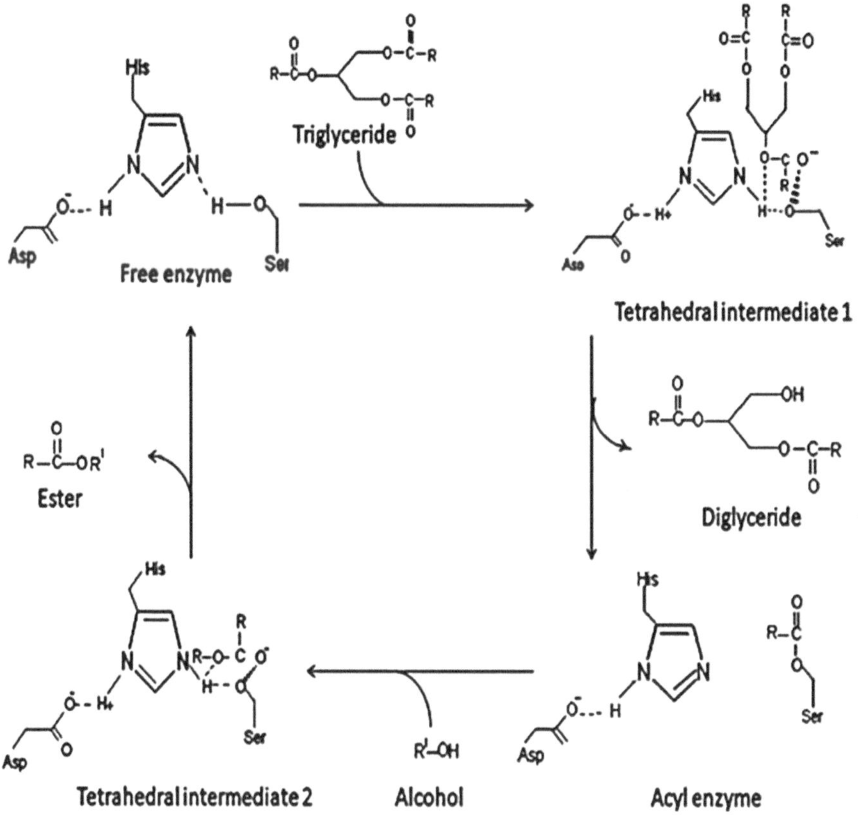

Fig. 2.8 Mechanism of lipase in transesterification (Jegannathan et al. 2008)

(aspartate and histidine) which hydrogen-bond to the oxyanion. Next, the electrons on the oxyanion are pushed back to the carbonyl carbon, and the proton currently on the histidine is transferred to the diglyceride, which is subsequently released (Al-Zuhair et al. 2007).

The serine ester formed reacts with alcohol to complete the transesterification. The histidine nitrogen removes hydrogen from the alcohol molecule forming the alkyl oxide anion. The hydroxide attacks the carbonyl carbon, the intermediate oxyanion is stabilized by a hydrogen bond (tetrahedral intermediate 2), the electrons are pushed back to the carbonyl carbon, and the free fatty acid is formed. The serine oxygen then reclaims the hydrogen situated on the histidine to re-establish the hydrogen-bonding network. The aspartic acid serves to pull positive charge from the histidine during the times it is fully protonated.

The immobilized lipases from various sources have been used in biodiesel production (see Table 2.6). Lipase from *Candida antarctica* has been selected by the majority of researchers. Other sources of enzyme used were produced from *Pseudomonas fluorescens, Burkholderia cepacia, Rhizomucor miehei, Chromobactrium viscosum, Porcine pancreas, and Thermomyces lanuginosus.* On the other hand, an interesting study by Turkan and Kalay (2006) on the elucidating mechanism of lipase for methanolysis of sunflower using three different immobilized lipases concludes that immobilized lipase from *Rhizomucor miehei* and *Thermomyces lanuginosus* catalyze the first step (conversion of triacylglyceride to diglyceride) of transesterification faster. Whereas, immobilized lipase from *Candida antarctica* catalyzes the second (di acylglyceride to mono acylglyceride) and third (monoacyl glyceride to acylester) steps faster. Turkan and Kalay (2006) suggested using a dual enzymatic system rather than the single lipase system in biodiesel production. The selection of lipase for immobilization to be used in biodiesel production depends on the process parameters of both immobilization and biodiesel production process. Therefore, screening of lipase suitable for process parameters is suggested.

2.4.4   Acyl Acceptors

Alcohol has been chosen as the acyl acceptors by the majority of the researchers (Table 2.3). Among alcohols, methanol and ethanol was popular. 2-butanol (Salis et al. 2005) and 2-propanol (Mukesh et al. 2006) were also reported as potential acyl acceptors. On the other hand methyl acetate (Du et al. 2005) and ethyl acetate (Mukesh et al. 2007) were also used as an acyl acceptor.

On the other hand, immobilized lipase has been found to be deactivated by lower linear alcohols. The degree of deactivation is inversely proportional to the number of carbon atoms in the linear lower alcohols (Chen and Wu 2003). Adding organic solvents have been adopted to overcome this problem. Nelson et al. (1996) used hexane to prevent the deactivation by a lower alcohol. Other solvents used include: Isooctane, Petroleum ether, 2-Propanol, Tetrahydrofuran and t-Butanol (Orcaire et al. 2006; Mittelbach 1990; Iso et al. 2001; Talukder et al. 2006; Rayon et al. 2007). Sung et al. (2007) explored the use of ionic liquids as solvents, whereas,

Table 2.7 Production of biodiesel using immobilized lipase by step wise addition of alcohol (Jegannathan et al. 2008)

Oil	Alcohol	A	B	C	D	E	Conversion in the 1st step %	Conversion in the 2nd step %	Conversion in the 3rd step %	References
Waste oil	Methanol	4	3	1/3	30	48	34 at 10 h	66 at 24 h	90.4 at 48	Watanabe et al. 2001
Soybean	Methanol	4	3	1/3	30	48	34 at 10 h	66 at 24 h	95.6 at 48	Watanabe et al. 2001
Soybean	Methanol	4	3	1/3	30	3.5	42.4 at 1 h	69.8 at 2.5 h	98.7 at 3.5 h	Samukawa et al. 2000
Soybean	Methanol	4	2	2/3	30	36	32 at 7 h	96.5 at 36 h		Watanabe et al. 2000
Soybean	Methanol	4	3	1/3	NA	NA	32 at 5 h	75 at 25 h	90 at 45 h	Du et al. 2005
Lard	Methanol	20	3	1/3	40	30	28 at 3 h	60 at 18 h	87.4 at 30 h	Lu et al. 2007

A: Percentage of immobilized lipase to the weight of oil
B: Number of methanol addition steps
C: Molar equivalent of alcohol in each step
D: Reaction temperature (°C)
E: Reaction time (h)

Oliveira and Oliveira (2001) reported the use of supercritical CO_2 use as a solvent. An advantage of using supercritical fluids, considering the complete process, was that after the system depressurization, a mixture of products and non-reacted substrate may be obtained without traces of solvent. However, the use of solvents is not recommended as it requires the addition of a solvent recovery unit and pressure unit which makes the production process costly.

Stepwise addition of alcohol was also used to get rid of the lipase deactivation by lower linear alcohols. The stepwise addition of alcohol has been discussed in detail (Shimada et al. 2002). A list of work reported on biodiesel production by immobilized lipase using step wise addition of alcohol is given in (Table 2.7). On the other hand, Talukder et al. (2007) used a salt-solution based controlled release system to control the concentration of methanol in the oil phase by dissolving methanol in $MgCl_2$ and LiCl salt solutions. Methanol was released according to its partitioning coefficient between the oil and the salt-solution phases. In addition it was reported that the glycerol produced during the process dissolves in the salt-solution phase, eliminating the glycerol deposition on the immobilized lipase. However, the use of salt solutions could generate more waste water and this could increase the production cost.

In the present scenario where production costs are given higher priority, the solvent free transesterification could be encouraged. Among the alcohols, the advantage of methanol as compared to higher alcohols is the fact that the two main products, glycerol and fatty acid methyl esters (FAME), are hardly miscible and thus form separate phases, an upper ester phase and a lower glycerol phase. This process removes glycerol from the reaction mixture and enables high conversion (Bacovsky et al. 2007). In addition, using methanol as an acyl acceptor for biodiesel production could be economical.

2.4.5   *Water Content*

Biocatalysts need minimum amount of water to retain their activity (Bommarius and Riebel-Bommarius 2000). Lipase has the unique feature of acting at the interface between an aqueous and an organic phase. Lipase interfacial action is due to the fact that their catalytic activity generally depends on the aggregation of the substrates. Activation of the enzymes involves unmasking and reconstructing the active site through conformational changes of the lipase molecule, which requires the presence of an oil-water interface. Lipase activity generally depends on the available interfacial area. With the addition of water, the amount of water available for oil to form oil–water droplets increases, thereby increasing the available interfacial area (Al-Zuhair et al. 2006). However, since lipases usually catalyze hydrolysis in aqueous media, excess water may also stimulate the competing hydrolysis reaction. The optimum water content is a compromise between minimizing hydrolysis and maximizing enzyme activity for the transesterification reaction (Noureddini et al. 2005).

Several researchers have reported the effect of water on biodiesel production (Table 2.3). With increased addition of water there was an increase in ester production. On the other hand few a researchers have reported that with the addition of water the ester production decreased (Shimada et al. 1999; Talukder et al. 2006). The amount of water to be maintained in biodiesel production using immobilized lipase depends on the feed stock (the water content of feed stock differs for waste oil to that of refined oil), source of lipase (some commercial lipase are in powder form which must be dissolved in coupling media before immobilization process), immobilization technique (some immobilization technique involves the use of water) and the type of acyl acceptor (analytical grade or reagent grade). Thus, it is recommended to optimize the water content depending on the reaction system used.

2.5   Immobilized Bioreactors and Operation Mode

Bioreactor is the heart of the manufacturing operation and the upstream and the downstream processes support this. The raw materials are prepared in the upstream section and the unconverted reactants, products, wastes are separated and purified and recyclable materials such as solvents recovered in the downstream section. A large number of biochemical reactor designs like agitated, sparged, and packed reactors are available, and the selection depends on the reaction kinetics, type of inhibition, mode of operation, aerobic or anaerobic type, whether the enzyme is in the native form or supported, physical properties of the biocell, the chemical and physical properties of the substrates used and the products formed, nature of gases formed, and the amount of heat to be removed or added (Mukesh et al. 2004).

2.5.1   Stirred Tank Bioreactor

Stirred vessels form the major workhorse in biochemical industry, many of them are operated batch wise and at a very large scale in a catalytic reaction involving enzymes. In order to make the process possible, the components have to be brought in contact at the molecular scale. In a typical reactor, the reacting species are added separately into the vessel in which reaction takes place, either as miscible or immiscible phases. The components from different streams are to be brought in intimate contact with each other if the reaction between them is to proceed. The reactor is, therefore, a three-dimensional space where these components are contacted with each other under either controlled conditions of temperature, pressure, etc.

When the reactants are miscible with each other or are present in the soluble form in a solvent, the reaction is said to be homogeneous. On the other hand, when the reactants are present in different phases, the system is heterogeneous. For a soluble enzyme-catalyzed reaction in aqueous phase where the substrate is also soluble, the reaction system is homogeneous. For an immobilized enzyme the system is heterogeneous with distinct liquid, solid, phases. Since in such heterogeneous conditions, the existence of transport processes across an interface characterizes the overall process, the relative rates of kinetic and transfer processes determine the rate-determining step (Mukesh et al. 2004). The stirred batch reactor is the type of reactor most commonly employed in bench scale and industrial scale applications (Pronk et al. 1988; Kang and Rhee 1989). Batch reactors are extremely versatile and easy to operate. Configuration includes glass flasks stirred with magnetic bars and vessels stirred by submerged impellers. In the case of the well-stirred batch reactor, sampling can be accomplished at a single, arbitrary located point.

2.5.2   Packed Bed Bioreactors

The packed bed reactor has traditionally been used for most large scale catalytic reactions because of its high efficiency, low cost, and ease of construction and operation. The packed bed reactor usually provides more surface area for reaction per unit volume If only a single liquid phase is employed, this phase may be pumped upward in order to reduce the tendency for bypassing of fluid or downward in order to take advantage of the driving force of gravity. There are two operational constraints which must be considered when operating packed bed reactor: (1) intra particle diffusion limitations on reaction rates; (2) high pressure drop across the reactor packing. External transport limitations are generally reduced in packed bed reactors by increasing the flow rates of the substrate through the column and changing the column reactor height-to-diameter ratio, thereby increasing the linear velocity.

Small particles are advantageous in reducing the effect of internal diffusion, but they increase the magnitude of any pressure drop. Regular-shaped particles are much better at reducing the problem of high-pressure drop in packed beds and of irregular flow pattern. In general, the size of the particle, which shows essentially no internal diffusion limitations, is so small that the pressure drops incurred become prohibitive (Ramachandra et al. 2002).

2.5.3   Operational Mode

In general there are three types of operation mode for immobilized enzyme reactions namely batch, continuous and fed batch mode. In literature, report on biodiesel production using immobilized lipase includes batch mode, continuous mode and fed batch mode in immobilized bioreactor.

2.5.4   Batch Mode

A batch mode has neither feed nor product streams. The substrates and biocatalyst are introduced at the start of the reaction, the reaction temperature and/or pressure raised in a pre-programmed manner, maintained at those conditions for a specified amount of time (or until the completion of the reaction), brought back to ambient conditions again in a pre-programmed manner, and finally the contents are discharged. The reactor is cleaned before the next batch is charged. Batch reactors have simple construction and are suitable for small production, but may lead to increased batch cycle time on account of downtime due to charging and discharging (Mukesh et al. 2004). A batch reactor could be a stirred tank reactor or a packed bed reactor.

2.5.5   Fed Batch Mode

In the fed batch mode, feed is introduced either continuously or intermittently while there is no continuous product removal. Similar to batch mode, A fed batch reactor could be a stirred tank reactor or a packed bed reactor. This type of mode is used in biodiesel production using immobilized lipase, where the methonol is added in stepwise addition (Watanabe et al. 2001; Samukawa et al. 2000; Du et al. 2005; Lu et al. 2007). Three and two step wise addition of methanol has been reported. The need for step wise addition was explained by the poisoning of immobilized lipase from some source organism by methanol. Production of biodiesel using immobilized lipase by step wise addition of alcohol is summarized in Table 2.7.

2.5.6 Continuous Mode

In the continuous mode, feed is introduced continuously or while there is continuous product removal. Similar to batch mode and fed batch mode could be a stirred tank reactor or a packed bed reactor. In biodiesel production using immobilized the lipase majority of the researchers selected batch operation in stirred tank immobilized bioreactor. The packed bed immobilized bioreactor has traditionally been used for most large scale catalytic reactors because of its high efficiency, low cost and ease of construction and operation (Malcata and Hill 1991). The mechanical stability and agglomeration of the immobilized enzyme must be considered when using a stirred tank immobilized bioreactor. Whereas, the pressure drop created across the immobilized bioreactor packing and the inter-particle diffusion limitations should be considered when using a packed bed immobilized bioreactor (Balcão et al. 1996).

On the other hand, Rayon et al. (2007), Halim et al. (2009) and Watanabe et al. (2000) used continuous fixed-bed reactors and reported the effect of flow rate on biodiesel production. However, in continuous packed bed reactor the glycerol produced during the reaction decreases the reaction rate of the immobilized lipase. Conversion could be enhanced if glycerol could be removed from the reaction mixture as the reaction proceeds (Watanabe et al. 2000). Glycerol formed during the reaction was separated continuously using a membrane reactor (Chen and Wu 2003; Be´lafi-bako et al. 2002). But, one of the limitations using membrane reactor might be their high cost compared to packed bed reactor and stirred tank reactor.

2.6 Kinetics of Biodiesel Production Using Immobilized Lipase

It is essential to understand the kinetics of the reaction to identify the optimal conditions for lipase catalyzed transesterification. Only a limited number of kinetic studies are found in the literature for biodiesel production using immobilized lipase. Most of the kinetic studies are described by the ping pong model with competitive inhibition by alcohol. Xu et al. (2005) reported the kinetics of lipase-catalyzed interesterification of soybean oil with methyl acetate for biodiesel production. A mechanism was proposed considering the presence of three consecutive reversible reactions. The rate constants for the three consecutive reactions from triacylglyceride to acyl ester were calculated and the results indicated that the first step reaction, triacylglyceride to diacylglyceride was the rate limiting step for the overall reaction. The proposed equations and the calculated rate constants are given in (Table 2.8). Dossat et al. (2002) proposed a model based on the ping pong bi with alcohol competitive inhibition mechanism to describe transesterification kinetics.

Al-Zuhair (2005) proposed a kinetic model for biodiesel production by two types of lipase, namely, *Rhizomucor miehei* lipase immobilized on ion-exchange resins and *Thermomyces antarctica* lipase immobilized on silica gel. There was a good

Table 2.8 Proposed kinetic models for biodiesel production using immobilized lipase (Jegannathan et al. 2008)

TG	Solvent	IL	Proposed kinetic equation	V_{max}	K_M	K_M [A]	K_i	References
SB	Methyl acetate	*Candida antarctica*	$Vi = Vmax\left[\dfrac{(A)(\rho mix - MA(A))MTG}{KmTG(A)\left(1+\dfrac{A}{Ki}\right) + (KmA+(A))(\rho mix - MA(A))/MTG}\right]$	1.9 Mol/Min	1 Mol/l	16 Mol/l	0.0455 Mol/l	Xu et al. 2005
SF	Butanol	*Rhizomucor miehei*	$Vi = \dfrac{Vmax(TG)}{1 + Ki[TG] + KTG[TG](1+[A]KIA) + KA\{A\}}$	250 mMol/ min.g	5.3 mM	55 mM	13 mM	Dossat et al. 2002
SF	Methanol	*Rhizomucor miehei*	$V = \dfrac{Vmax(TG)}{1 + Ki[TG] + KTG[TG](1+[A]KIA) + KA[A]}$	0.414 Mol/ min	0.16 Mol/cm^3	0.98×10^{-4} Mol/ cm^3	1.9 Mol/ cm^3	Al-Zuhair 2005
WCP	Methanol	*Candida antarctica*	$Vi = \dfrac{Vmax(TG)(A)}{Km[TG][A] + \left(1+\dfrac{[A]}{Ki[A]}\right) + KmA[TG] + [TG][A]}$	2.34 M min^{-1}	2.61 M	10.25 M	1.60 M	Halim and Kamaruddin 2008

TG (Triglyceride) A (Alcohol) SB (Soybean oil) SF (Sunflower oil) WCP (Waste cooking palm oil)
IL (Immobilized lipase) K_m [TG] (Apparent Michaelis-Menten constant for triglycerides)
K_m[A] (Apparent Michaelis-Menten constant for methyl acetate or alcohol) V_i (Initial reaction rate)
V_{max} (The initial maximum velocity of reaction) K_i (Inhibition Constant)

agreement between the experimental results of the initial rate of reaction and those predicted by the proposed model equations, for both enzymes. The proposed model equation (Table 2.8) can be used to predict the rate of methanolysis of vegetable oils in a batch or a continuous reaction. Similarly, Halim and Kamaruddin (2008) had proposed a Ping Pong kinetic model with alcohol inhibition for the biodiesel production from waste cooking palm oil using immobilized lipase (Novozyme 435). The kinetic parameters and the model equation are given in Table 2.8. In enzymatic reaction systems, the Michaelis Menten mechanism and the performance equation of batch reactor (Kayode Coker 2001) can also be used to estimate the kinetic parameters. This approach has been attempted in the biodiesel production using immobilized lipase elsewhere.

From the literature discussed in the above sections it is clear that no attempt has been made so far to use carrageenan as a matrix for lipase immobilization in biodiesel production. Nowadays, the biotechnological production of biodiesel with lipases has received great consideration and is undergoing a rapid development. This is understandable since the trend towards ecologically acceptable processes is steadily growing (Shimada et al. 2002). Hence it is expected that the future research work of biodiesel production using immobilized lipase should focus on environmental benign matrix and an immobilization method with milder process conditions.

2.7 Carrageenan as a Matrix for Lipase Immobilization

The choice of immobilization method and the support depends on the nature of the biocatalyst, the process conditions, the type of reactor to be used, and the specific application of the biocatalyst. In general, the important characteristics are operational stability, particle size, solubility (or insolubility), biodegradability, diffusivity of substrates and/or reactants (Velde and Ruiter 2002). These characteristics can be achieved by immobilizing enzyme in carrageenan matrix.

κ-carrageenan is a naturally occurring polysaccharide isolated from a marine red algae. It is readily available, cheap and non-toxic polymer composed of repeating units of β-d-galactose sulfate and 3, 6-anhydro-d-galactose units. Several types of carrageenans differ in the number and position of sulphate groups. The most common types of carrageenan are traditionally identified by a Greek prefix. The three commercially most important carrageenans are called, ι, κ, and λ-carrageenan. ι and κ-carrageenans are gel-forming, whereas λ-carrageenan is a thickener/ viscosity builder and, therefore, not applicable for immobilization techniques. The gel-forming ι and κ-carrageenans are composed of alternating, 3-linked β-d-galactopyranose and 4-linked 3, 6-anhydro- α-D-galactopyranose units, forming the disaccharide repeating unit or diad of the carrageenans (Fig. 2.9) (Velde and Ruiter 2002). The sources of gelling carrageenans seem to be *Eucheuma cottonii* (Kappaphycus alvarezii) and *Eucheuma spinosum* (Piculell 2006).

Gel formation is the most important feature of carrageenan and essential for their application in immobilization techniques. In general terms, ι-carrageenan forms

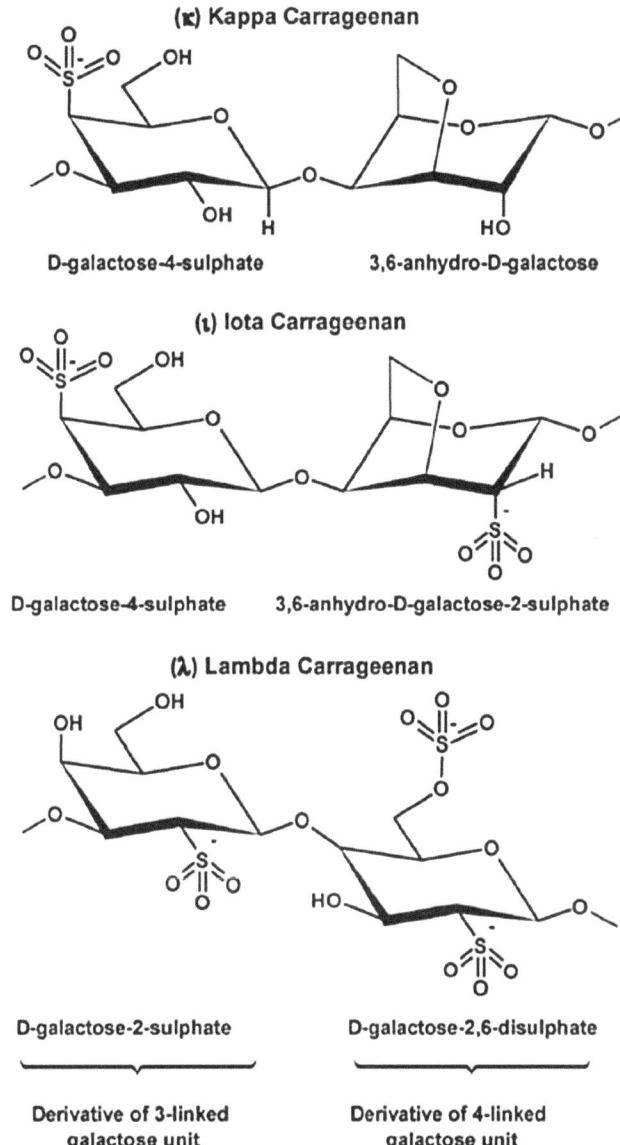

Fig. 2.9 Structures of different types of carrageenan (Sankalia et al. 2006)

soft and weak gels that are freeze/thaw stable, whereas κ-carrageenan gels are hard, strong, and brittle gels that are freeze/thaw instable. Hence κ-carrageenan is a suitable support material for the immobilization as proven by several applications in different industrial processes. κ-carrageenan as matrix for enzyme immobilization in different application is summarized in Table 2.9 (Velde and Ruiter 2002).

Table 2.9 Overview of applications of enzymes immobilized in carrageenan matrices (Velde and Ruiter 2002)

Enzyme	Application	Method
Aminoacylase	Immobilisation studies	Droplet, gel
Aspartase	Immobilisation studies	Droplet, gel
Catalase	Hydrogen peroxide determination	Dehydration
Choline oxidase	butyrylcholinesterase Analysis of organophosphorus pesticides	Dehydration
Choline oxidase	phospholipase D Lecithin analysis in food and drugs	Dehydration
Esterase	Transesterification of 3-phenylglutamic acid esters	Droplet, gel
Fumarase	Immobilization studies	Droplet, gel
Galactosidase	Hydrolysis of lactose	Droplet
Glucoamylase	Ethanol production from corn starch	Droplet
Lipase	Esterification of laurate to propyl laurate	Emulsion
Naringinase	Debittering of citrus juice	Droplet
Subtilisin	Transesterification of N-acetyl phenylalanine esters	Dehydration
Proteases	Production of casein hydrolysates	Droplet, gel
Tannase	Hydrolysis of tea tannins	Droplet
Tyrosinase	Monitoring the rancification process of olive oils	Dehydration
Acetylcholinesterase	Immobilization studies	Droplet, gel
Lipase	hydrolysis of olive oil	Droplet, gel
Lipase	esterification in isooctane	Emulsion, gel
Amylase	Immobilization studies	Droplet, gel
Chymotrypsin	Immobilization studies	Droplet, gel

2.8 Methods for Biocatalyst Immobilization in Carrageenan

The techniques for the immobilization of biocatalysts into carrageenan are facilitated by the fact that under non-gelling conditions carrageenan solutions exhibit moderate viscosity and are relatively easy to handle. Gelling is promoted by lowering the temperature or by the addition of gel inducing agents. In the literature the immobilization techniques for enzyme immobilization using carrageenan as matrix falls under the general method of entrapment. The techniques can be roughly divided into four groups: gel method, droplet method, emulsion method, and dehydration method. These four methods are described below.

2.8.1 Gel Method

The simplest immobilization technique is the gel method. An aqueous solution of carrageenan is heated above the gel temperature of the carrageenan. After dissolution of the carrageenan the solution is mixed with an enzyme solution and the mixture is allowed to cool and gel. The gel is then cut into the desired shape, such as cubes or crushed into small particles. The advantage of this method is the fact that the gels can be produced in any shape.

2.8.2   Droplet Method

The droplet method is widely used for the preparation of spherical gel beads. In contrast to the gel and emulsion method, for this approach the carrageenan/ biocatalyst mixture requires no heating and can be prepared at room temperature. The carrageenan is dissolved in distilled water and mixed with a solution or suspension of the bioactive material, resulting in a solution/suspension of low ionic strength and moderate viscosity. This solution/suspension is extruded drop wise into a stirred potassium chloride solution using techniques such as, a pump with a needle, a syringe, or a nozzle. Under these conditions the carrageenan solution immediately solidifies (Velde and Ruiter 2002).

2.8.3   Emulsion Method

In this method an aqueous solution/suspension of carrageenan and biocatalyst is heated above the gel temperature. This aqueous phase is then mixed with a heated, non-reactive food-grade oil phase (canola oil or soybean oil has been used in the above-mentioned examples). The two phases are vigorously mixed to obtain biocatalysts/carrageenan droplets of the desired size. Under continuous stirring the droplets are gelled by lowering the temperature of the oil. The oil is then decanted from the resulting beads and the beads are washed with appropriate buffer and/or salt solutions. By controlling the stirring rate the desired particular size is obtained (Velde and Ruiter 2002).

2.8.4   Dehydration Method

In this method first the carrageenan beads or films are prepared without enzyme by the above-mentioned droplet method. Prepared carrageenan beads or films are dehydrated, either by drying or lyophilisation. Immersing or suspending the dehydrated gels in an aqueous solution of enzymes results in swelling of the gel beads or films and embedding of the enzyme material.

Table 2.9 summarizes the immobilization method employed for different enzymes in carrageenan matrix. No attempt has yet been made to immobilize enzyme in κ-carrageenan by encapsulation method. Similarly no attempt has been made to use κ-carrageenan as a matrix for lipase immobilization in biodiesel production.

Hence study of lipase encapsulation in κ-carrageenan would be a new and biodiesel production using κ-carrageenan encapsulated lipase would be an ecofreindly approach and would reduce the environmental impact further comparing to the current available biodiesel production process (Velde and Ruiter 2002).

2.9 LCA Studies on Biodiesel Production

There are only few literature available reporting the life cycle assessment of biodiesel production. Harding et al. 2008 has compared the life cycle assessment of biodiesel production from rape seed using alkali catalyst, immobilized enzyme catalyst, and alcohols (methanol and ethanol). The study reveals that enzyme catalysed biodiesel production has environmental advantages due to avoided use of chemical catalyst and neutralizing acid. The lower pressures and temperatures obtained help to give more favourable LCA results and all environmental impacts considered are reduced compared to the alkali catalyst. Whereas, using methanol has higher impact on environment than the ethanol (Harding et al. 2008). However, the immobilized enzyme considered in this study was a commercial enzyme. Hence the detail study of enzyme production process involved was not included in the inventory analysis.

The environmental impact of biodiesel production from crude palm and refined palm oil using conventional chemical catalyst was compared with the catalyst free supercritical process in a recent study by Kiwjaroun et al. (2009). It was concluded that for both crude palm oil and refined palm oil, the supercritical process always generated a higher impact on the environment, because of its requirement for large amounts of methanol during the reaction and consequently the energy expenditure in methanol recirculation in the recycle loop.

In a recent study Yee et al. (2009) compared the life cycle assessment of biodiesel production from palm oil with rapeseed oil. From this study, it was found that the utilization of palm biodiesel would generate an energy yield ratio of 3.53 (output energy/input energy), indicating a net positive energy. The energy ratio for palm biodiesel was found to be more than double the ratio for rapeseed biodiesel, which was only at 1.44. This indicates that palm oil would be a more sustainable feedstock for biodiesel production as compared to rapeseed oil. In terms of green house gas assessment, it has been concluded that the production of palm and rapeseed biodiesel brings no negative impact to the environment as the amount of CO_2 emitted to the atmosphere is much lower than the CO_2 absorbed from the atmosphere. Also, the emission of CO_2 per litre from the combustion of biodiesel is 38 % less than that of petrol. Contrary to some reports which challenge the sustainability of palm oil as an environment-friendly source of energy, the results of this LCA study has shown that palm diesel has the potential to become the major renewable energy in the future, with huge positive energy ratio and significant reduction in CO_2 emission.

Table 2.10   LCA studies on biodiesel production

Goal of the LCA study	Method that show less impact on environment	References
Comparison between inorganic and biological catalysis for the production of rape seed biodiesel	Biological catalyst	Harding et al. 2008
Comparison of palm biodiesel and rapeseed biodiesel production using alkaline catalyst	Palm oil	Yee et al. 2009
Comparison of alkaline catalyst palm biodiesel and supercritical methanol palm biodiesel	Alkaline catalyst	Kiwjaroun et al. 2009

The LCA results have been summarized in the Table 2.10. From the table in can be concluded that production of biodiesel from palm oil using immobilized catalyst would have less environmental impact.

2.10   Economical Assessment of Biodiesel Production

In the literature, most of the economic assessment studies conducted on biodiesel production are mainly evaluated based on continuous processes. The costs involved in the production of 8,000 to 125,000 tonnes/year of biodiesel for a continuous supercritical methanol process involving waste cooking oil was estimated by Kasteren and Nisworo (2007). Whereas, West et al. (2008) assessed the costs involved in producing 8,000 tonne/year of biodiesel for four processes involving waste cooking oil; (1) a continuous homogeneous alkali-catalyzed process, (2) a continuous homogeneous acid-catalyzed process, (3) a continuous heterogeneous acid-catalyzed process and (4) a continuous supercritical methanol process.

Similarly, You et al. (2008) evaluated the costs involved in the production of 8,000–100,000 tonnes/year of biodiesel for a continuous homogeneous alkali-catalyzed process involving soybean oil. Marchetti and Errazu (2008) assessed the costs involved in producing 36,036 tonnes/year of biodiesel for the same four processes. In these both four processes, the continuous heterogeneous acid-catalyzed process had the lowest manufacturing costs. Recently Sakai et al. (2009) assessed the homogeneous and heterogeneous alkali-catalyzed batch processes for a biodiesel production ranging from 1,452 tonnes/year (5,000 l/day) to 14,520 tonnes/year (50,000 l/day). KOH as a homogeneous catalyst and CaO as a heterogeneous catalyst were selected for evaluation. A comparison of all the studies conducted on biodiesel cost assessment using different catalytic process is given in the Table 2.11. However, the biodiesel production using heterogeneous enzyme in batch processes is not evaluated. Thus evaluating the economics of biodiesel production using immobilized catalyst would provide new information.

Table 2.11 Comparison between previous studies for biodiesel production plants economic assessment (Sakai et al. 2009)

Plant capacity (tonne/year)	Process type	Catalyst	Oil	Glycerol credit $/tonne	Manufacturing cost[a] $/tonne[b]	Fixed cost $/tonne	Plant cost $ million	References
8,000	Continuous	None[c]	Waste cooking oil	127	442	290	2.00[d]	Kasteren and Nisworo 2007
125,000	Continuous	None[c]	Waste cooking oil	127	150	21	10.40[d]	
8,000	Continuous	Homogenous alkali	Soybean oil	380	685	118	1.35	You et al. 2008
30,000	Continuous	Homogenous alkali	Soybean oil	380	582	68	4.04	
100,000	Continuous	Homogenous alkali	Soybean oil	380	547	50	11.67	
8,000	Continuous	Homogenous alkali	Waste cooking oil	73	526	75	1.59	West et al. 2008
8,000	Continuous	Homogenous acid	Waste cooking oil	76	485	81	1.99	
8,000	Continuous	Heterogenous acid	Waste cooking oil	71	386	59	0.63	
8,000	Continuous	None[c]	Waste cooking oil	75	459	83	2.15	
36,036	Continuous	Homogenous alkali	Waste cooking oil	74	423	49	7.42[d]	Marchetti, and Errazu 2008
36,036	Continuous	Homogenous alkali	Waste cooking oil	71	439	40	7.33[d]	
36,036	Continuous	Homogenous acid	Waste cooking oil	99	425	31	5.15[d]	
36,036	Continuous	Heterogenous acid	Waste cooking oil	67	918	36	8.44[d]	
7,260	Batch	Homogenous alkali	Waste cooking oil	0	598	194	6.48[d]	Sakai et al. 2009
7,260	Batch	Homogenous alkali	Waste cooking oil	0	641	225	7.99[d]	
7,260	Batch	Heterogenous acid	Waste cooking oil	0	584	200	6.76[d]	
7,260	Batch	Heterogenous acid	Waste cooking oil	0	622	232	8.30[d]	

[a]Manufacturing cost = Variable cost + fixed cost − glycerol credit, not includes general expenses
[b]Based on tonne-FAME
[c]Supercritical methanol process
[d]Includes utility equipment

References

Akoh CC, Chang SS, Lee GG, Shaw JJ (2007) Enzymatic approach to biodiesel production. J Agric Food Chem 55:8995–9005

Al-Zuhair S (2005) Production of biodiesel by lipase-catalyzed transesterification of vegetable Oils: a kinetics study. Biotechnol Prog 21:1442–1448

Al-Zuhair S, Fan YW, Lim SJ (2007) Proposed kinetic mechanism of the production of biodiesel from palm oil using lipase. Process Biochem 42:951–960

Al-Zuhair S, Jayaraman KS, Smita K, Chan W (2006) The effect of fatty acid concentration and water content on the production of biodiesel by lipase. Biochem Eng J 30:212–217

Al-zuhair S (2007) Production of biodiesel: possibilities and challenges. Biofuel Bioprod Bior 1:57–66

Bacovsky D, Körbitz W, Mittelbach M, Wörgetter M (2007) Biodiesel production: technologies and European providers. IEA Task 39 Report T39-B6

Balcão VM, Paiva AL, Malcata FX (1996) Bioreactors with immobilized lipases: state of the art. Enzyme Microb Technol 18:392–416

Be´Lafi-Bako K, Kova´Cs F, Gubicza L, Hancsok J (2002) Enzymatic biodiesel production from sunflower oil by *Candida antarctica* lipase in a solvent-free system. Biocatal Biotransfor 20:437–439

Bommarius AS, Riebel-Bommarius BR (2000) Biocatalysts: fundamentals and applications. John Wiley & sons, New York

Bondioli P (2004) The preparation of fatty acid esters by means of catalytic reactions. Top Catal 27:77–82

Bonrath W, Karge R, Netscher T (2002) Lipase-catalyzed transformations as key-steps in the large-scale preparation of vitamins. J Mol Catal B: Enzym 19:67–72

Bosley JA, Peilow AD (1997) Immobilization of lipase on porous polypropylene: reduction in esterification efficiency at low loading. J Am Oil Chem Soc 74:107–111

Canakci M, Gerpen VJ (2001) Biodiesel production from oils and fats with high free fatty acids. Trans ASAE 44:1429–1436

Cao LQ, Langen VL, Sheldon RA (2003) Immobilized enzymes: carrier-bound or carrier-free? Curr Opin Biotechnol 14:387–394

Cao L (2005) Immobilized enzymes: science or art? Curr Opin Chem Biol 9:217 226

Caye MD, Nghiem PN, Terry HW (2008) Biofuels engineering process technology. McGraw-Hill, New York

Cecilia GA, Amalia AC, Ferreira M (2007) Relation between lipase structures and their catalytic ability to hydrolyse triglycerides and phospholipids. Enzyme Microb Technol 41:35–43

Chamorro S, Sanchez-Montero JM, Alcantara AR, Sinisterra JV (1998) Treatment of *Candida rugosa* lipase with short-chain polar organic solvents enhances its hydrolytic and synthetic activities. Biotechnol Lett 20:499–505

Chen JW, Wu WT (2003) Regeneration of immobilized Candida antarctica Lipase for transesterification. J Biosci Bioeng 95:466–469

Chisti Y (2007) Biodiesel from microalgae. Biotechnol Adv 25:294–306

Colton IJ, Ahmed SN, Kazlauskas RJ (1995) A2-propanol treatment increases the enantioselectivity of Candida rugosa lipase toward esters of chiral carboxylic acids. J Org Chem 60:212–217

Concawe (2006) Well-to-wheels analysis of future automotive fuels and power trains in the European context, European commission. EUCAR and EC Joint Research Centre. Report. (http://ies.jrc.ec.europa.eu/wtw.html)

Diasakou M, Louloudi A, Papayannakos N (1998) Kinetics of the noncatalytic transesterification of soybean oil. Fuel 77:1297–1302

Dizge N, Aydiner C, Derya YI, Mahmut B, Aziz T, Keskinler B (2009) Biodiesel production from sunflower, soybean, and waste cooking oils by transesterification using lipase immobilized onto a novel microporous polymer. Bioresour Technol 100:1983–1991

Dong HL, Jung MK, Seong WK, Ji WL, Seung WK (2006) Pretreatment of lipase with soybean oil before immobilization to prevent loss of activity. Biotechnol Lett 28:1965–1969

Dossat V, Combes D, Marty A (2002) Lipase-catalyzed transesterification of high oleic sunflower oil. Enzyme Microb Technol 30:90–94

Du W, Xu Y, Liu D, Zeng J (2004) Comparative study on lipase-catalyzed transformation of soybean oil for biodiesel production with different acyl acceptors. J Mol Catal B: Enzym 30:25–129

Du W, Xu Y, Liu D, Li Z (2005) Study on acyl migration in immobilized lipozyme TL-catalyzed transesterification of soybean oil for biodiesel production. J Mol Catal B: Enzym 37:68–71

Fjerbaek L, Christensen KV, Norddahl B (2009) A review of the current State of biodiesel production using enzymatic transesterification. Biotechnol Bioeng 102:1298–1315

Freedman BW, Kwolek F, Pryde EH (1986) Quantitation in the analysis of transesterified soybean oil by capillary gas chromatography. J Am Oil Chem Soc 63:1370–1375

Halim SFA, Kamaruddin AH (2008) Catalytic studies of lipase on FAME production from waste cooking palm oil in a tert-butanol system. Process Biochem 43:1436–1439

Halim SFA, Kamaruddin AH, Fernando WJN (2009) Continuous biosynthesis of biodiesel from waste cooking palm oil in a packed bed reactor: optimization using response surface methodology (RSM) and mass transfer studies. Bioresour Technol 100:710–716

Harding KG, Dennis JS, Blottnitz HV, Harrison STL (2008) A life-cycle comparison between inorganic and biological catalysis for the production of biodiesel. J Clean Prod 16:1368–1378

Hsu A, Jones K, Marmer WN, Foglia TA (2001) Production of alkyl esters from tallow and grease using lipase immobilized in a phyllosilicate sol-gel. J Am Oil Chem Soc 78:585–588

International Energy Agency (2007) Energy technology essentials: biomass for power generation and CHP. Report

Iso M, Chen B, Eguchi M, Kudo T, Shrestha S (2001) Production of biodiesel fuel from triglycerides and alcohol using immobilized lipase. J Mol Catal B: Enzym 16:53–58

Jegannathan KR, Abang S, Poncelet D, Chan ES, Ravindra P (2008) Production of biodiesel using immobilized lipase- a critical review. Crit Rev Biotechnol 28:253–264

Jegannathan KR, Chan ES, Ravindra P (2009) Harnessing biofuels: a global renaissance in energy production? Renew Sust Energy Rev 13:2163–2168

Kang ST, Rhee JS (1989) Characteristics of immobilized lipase-catalyzed hydrolysis of olive oil of high concentration in reverse phase systems. Biotechnol Bioeng 33:1469–1476

Karube I, Yugeta Y, Suzuki S (1977) Electric field control of lipase membrane activity. Biotechnol Bioeng 19:1493–1501

Kasteren VJMN, Nisworo AP (2007) A process model to estimate the cost of industrial scale biodiesel production from waste cooking oil by supercritical transesterification. Resour Conserv Recycle 50:442–458

Kayode Coker A (2001) Modeling of chemical kinetics and reactor design. Gulf Publishing Company, Houston

Kennedy JF, Melo EHM, Jumel K (1990) Immobilized enzymes end cells. Chem Eng Prog 86:81–89

Kiwjaroun C, Tubtimdee C, Piumsomboon P (2009) LCA studies comparing biodiesel synthesized by conventional and supercritical methanol methods. J Clean Prod 17:143–153

Kreiner M, Parker MC, Barry DM (2001) Enzyme-coated micro-crystals: a 1-step method for high activity biocatalyst preparation. Chem Commun 12:1096–1097

Kumari V, Shah S, Gupta MN (2007) Preparation of biodiesel by lipase-catalyzed transesterification of high free fatty acid containing oil from *Madhuca indica*. Energy Fuel 21:368–372

Kusdiana D, Saka S (2001) Methyl esterification of free fatty acids of rapeseed oil as treated in supercritical methanol. J Chem Eng Japan 34:383–387

Li L, Du W, Liu D, Wang L, Li Z (2006) Lipase catalyzed transesterification of rapeseed oils for biodiesel production with a novel organic solvents as the reaction medium. J Mol Catal B: Enzym 43:58–62

Licht FO (2008) World ethanol & biofuels. Report, no. 16

López DE, Goodwin JG, Bruce DA (2007) Transesterification of triacetin with methanol on nafion acid resins. J Catal 245:379–385

Lu J, Nie K, Xie F, Wang F, Tan T (2007) Enzymatic synthesis of fatty acids methyl esters from lard with immobilized Candida sp. 99–125. Process Biochem 42:1367–1370

Malcata FX, Hill CG (1991) Use of a lipase immobilized in a membrane reactor to hydrolyze the glycerides of butter oil. Biotechnol Bioeng 38:853–868

Marchetti JM, Errazu AF (2008) Technoeconomic study of supercritical biodiesel production plant. Energy Conver Manag 49:2160–2164

Mittelbach M, Worgetter M, Pernkopf J, Junek H (1983) Diesel fuel derived from vegetable oils: preparation and use of rape oil methyl-ester. Energy Agric 2:369–384

Mittelbach M (1990) Lipase catalyzed alcoholysis of sunflower oil. J Am Oil Chem Soc 67: 168–170

Mittelbach M, Remschmidt C (2006) Biodiesel: the comprehensive handbook. Martin Mittelbach, Graz

Mukesh D, Anil Kumar K, Gaikar VG (2004) Biotransformations and bioprocesses. Marcel Dekker, New York

Mukesh KM, Reddy JRC, Rao BVSK, Prasad RBN (2006) Lipase-mediated transformation of vegetable oils into biodiesel using propan-2-ol as acyl acceptor. Biotechnol Lett 28:637–640

Mukesh KM, Reddy JRC, Rao BVSK, Prasad RBN (2007) Lipase-mediated conversion of vegetable oils into biodiesel using ethyl acetate as acyl acceptor. Bioresour Technol 98:1260–1264

Nelson LA, Foglia TA, Marmer WN (1996) Lipase-catalyzed production of biodiesel. J Am Oil Chem Soc 73:1191–1195

Nie K, Xie F, Wang T, Tan T (2006) Lipase catalyzed methanolysis to produce biodiesel: optimization of the biodiesel production. J Mol Catal B: Enzym 43:142–147

Noureddini H, Gao X, Philkana RS (2005) Immobilized *Pseudomonas cepacia* lipase for biodiesel fuel production from soybean oil. Bioresour Technol 96:769–777

Oliveira JV, Oliveira D (2001) Enzymatic alcoholysis of palm kernel oil in n-hexane and $SCCO_2$. J Supercrit Fluid 19:141–148

Orcaire O, Buisson P, Pierre AC (2006) Application of silica aerogel encapsulated lipases in the synthesis of biodiesel by transesterification reactions. J Mol Catal B: Enzym 42:106–113

Piculell L (2006) Gelling carrageenans, food polysaccharides and their applications, 2nd edn. Taylor & Francis, London

Pleiss J, Fisher M, Schmid RD (1998) Anatomy of lipase binding sites: the scissile fatty acid binding site. Chem Phys 93:67–80

Posorske LH (1984) Industrial-Scale application of enzymes to the fats and oil industry. J Am Oil Chem Soc 61:1758–1760

Pronk W, Kerkhof PJA, Van Helden C, Vant Reit K (1988) The hydrolysis of triglycerides by immobilized lipase in a hydrophilic membrane reactor. Biotechnol Bioeng 32:512–518

Ramachandra MV, Jayadev B, Muniswaran PKA (2002) Hydrolysis of oils by using immobilized lipase enzyme: a review. Biotechnol Bioproc Eng 7:57–66

Rayon D, Daz M, Ellenrieder G, Locatelli S (2007) Enzymatic production of biodiesel from cotton seed oil using t-butanol as a solvent. Bioresour Technol 98:648–653

Reyed M (2007) Novel hybrid entrapment approach for probiotic cultures and its application during lyophilization. Internet J Biol Anthr 3: 2.

REN21 (2009) Renewables Global Status Report: Update

Sakai T, Kawashima A, Koshikawa T (2009) Economic assessment of batch biodiesel production processes using homogeneous and heterogeneous alkali catalysts. Bioresour Technol 100:3268–3276

Salis A, Pinna M, Monduzzi M, Solinas V (2005) Biodiesel production from triolein and short chain alcohols through biocatalysis. J Biotechnol 119:291–299

Samukawa T, Kaieda M, Matsumoto T, Ban K, Kondo A, Shimada Y, Noda H, Fukuda H (2000) Pretreatment of immobilized *Candida antarctica* lipase for biodiesel fuel production from plant oil. J Biosci Bioeng 90:180–183

Sankalia MG, Mashru RC, Sankalia MJ, Sutariya VB (2006) Stability improvement of alpha-amylase entrapped in kappa-carrageenan beads: physicochemical characterization and optimization using composite index. Int J Pharm 312:1–14

Shah S, Sharma S, Gupta MN (2004) Biodiesel preparation by lipase-catalyzed transesterification of Jatropha oil. Energy Fuel 18:154–159

Shah S, Gupta MN (2006) Lipase catalyzed preparation of biodiesel from Jatropha oil in a solvent free system. Process Biochem 42:409–414

Sheehan J, Cambreco V, Duffield J, Garboski M, Shapouri H (1998) An overview of biodiesel and petroleum diesel life cycles. A report by US Department of Agriculture and Energy 1–35

Shimada Y, Watanabe Y, Samukawa T (1999) Conversion of vegetable oil to biodiesel using immobilized *Candida antarctica* lipase. J Am Oil Chem Soc 76:789–793

Shimada Y, Watanabe H, Sugihara A, Tominaga Y (2002) Enzymatic alcoholysis for biodiesel fuel production and application of the reaction to oil processing. J Mol Catal B: Enzym 17:133–142

Soumanou MM, Bornscheuer UT (2003) Improvement in lipase-catalyzed synthesis of fatty acid methyl esters from sunflower oil. Enzyme Microb Technol 33:97–103

Sriappareddy T, Shinji H, Takanori T, Talukder MR, Kondo A, Fukuda H (2007) Immobilized recombinant Aspergillus oryzae expressing heterologous lipase: an efficient whole-cell biocatalyst for enantioselective transesterification in non-aqueous medium. J Mol Catal B: Enzym 48:33–37

Sriappareddy T, Talukder MR, Hama S, Numata T, Kondo A, Fukuda H (2008) Enzymatic production of biodiesel from Jatropha oil: a comparative study of immobilized-whole cell and commercial lipases as a biocatalyst. Biochem Eng J 39:185–189

Srivastava A, Prasad R (2000) Triglycerides-based diesel fuels. Renew Sustain Energy Rev 4:111–113

Svendsen A (2000) Lipase protein engineering. Biochim Biophys Acta 1543:223–238

Sung HH, Lan MN, Lee SN, Hwang SM, Koo YM (2007) Lipase-catalyzed biodiesel production from soybean oil in ionic liquids. Enzyme Microb Technol 41:480–483

Talukder MMR, Beatrice KLM, Song OP, Puah S, Wu JC, Won CJ, Chow Y (2007) Improved method for efficient production of biodiesel production from palm oil. Biocatal Biotransfor 22:141–144

Talukder MMR, Puah SM, Wu JC, Won CJ, Chow Y (2006) Lipase-catalyzed methanolysis of palm oil in presence and absence of organic solvent for production of biodiesel. Biocatal Biotransfor 24:257–262

Tillman D, Hill J, Lehman C (2006) Carbon-negative biofuels from low input high-diversity grassland biomass. Science 314:1598–1600

Turkan A, Kalay S (2006) Monitoring lipase- catalyzed methanolysis of sunflower oil by reversed-phase high-performance liquid chromatography: elucidation of the mechanism of lipases. J Chromatogr A 1127:34–44

Velde FV, Ruiter GAD (2002) Polysaccharides II: polysaccharides from eukaryotes. Wiley-VCH, Weinheim

Wang L, Du W, Liu D, Li L, Dai N (2006) Lipase-catalyzed biodiesel production from soybean oil deodorizer distillate with absorbent present in tert-butanol system. J Mol Catal B: Enzym 43:29–32

Watanabe Y, Shimada Y, Sugihara A, Noda H, Fukuda H, Tominaga Y (2000) Continuous production of biodiesel fuel from vegetable oil using immobilized Candida antarctica Lipase. J Am Oil Chem Soc 77:355–360

Watanabe Y, Shimada Y, Sugihara A, Tominaga Y (2001) Enzymatic conversion of waste edible oil to biodiesel fuel in a fixed-bed bioreactor. J Am Oil Chem Soc 78:703–707

West AH, Posarac D, Ellis N (2008) Assessment of four biodiesel production processes using HYSYS plant. Bioresour Technol 99:6587–6601

Wu WH, Foglia TA, Marmer WN, Phillips JG (1999) Optimizing production of ethyl esters of grease using 95 % ethanol by response surface methodology. J Am Oil Chem Soc 76:517–521

Xavier MF, Hector RR, Hugo SG, Charles GH, Clyde HA (1990) Immobilized lipase reactors for modification of fats and oils- a review. J Am Oil Chem Soc 67:890–910

Xu Y, Du W, Liu D, Zeng J (2003) A novel enzymatic route for biodiesel production from renewable oils in a solvent-free medium. Biotechnol Lett 25:1239–1241

Xu Y, Du W, Liu D (2005) Study on the kinetics of enzymatic interesterification of triglycerides for biodiesel production with methyl acetate as the acyl acceptor. J Mol Catal B: Enzym 32:241–245

Yadav GD, Jadhav SR (2005) Synthesis of reusable lipases by immobilization on hexagonal meso-porous silica and encapsulation in calcium alginate: transesterification in non-aqueous medium. Micropor Mesopor Mat 86:215–222

Yagiz F, Kazan D, Akin AN (2007) Biodiesel production from waste oils by using lipase immobi-lized on hydrotalcite and zeolites. Chem Eng J 134:262–267

Yang G, Tian-Wei T, Kai-Li N, Fang W (2006) Immobilization of lipase on macroporous resin and its application in synthesis of biodiesel in low aqueous media. Chin J Biotechnol 22:114–118

Yazdani SS, Gonzalez R (2007) Anaerobic fermentation of glycerol: a path to economic viability for the biofuels industry. Curr Opin Biotechnol 18:213–21

Yee KF, Tan KT, Abdullah AZ, Lee KT (2009) Life cycle assessment of palm biodiesel: revealing facts and benefits for sustainability. Appl Energy 86:189–196

Yesiloglu Y (2004) Immobilized lipase-catalyzed ethanolysis of sunflower oil. J Am Oil Chem Soc 81:157–160

You YD, Shie JL, Chang CY, Huang SH, Pai CY, Yu YH, Chang CH (2008) Economic cost analysis of biodiesel production: case in soybean oil. Energy Fuel 22:182–189

Zeng HG, Liao K, Deng X, Jiang H, Zhang F (2009) Characterization of the lipase immobilized on Mg–Al hydrotalcite for biodiesel. Process Biochem 44:791–798

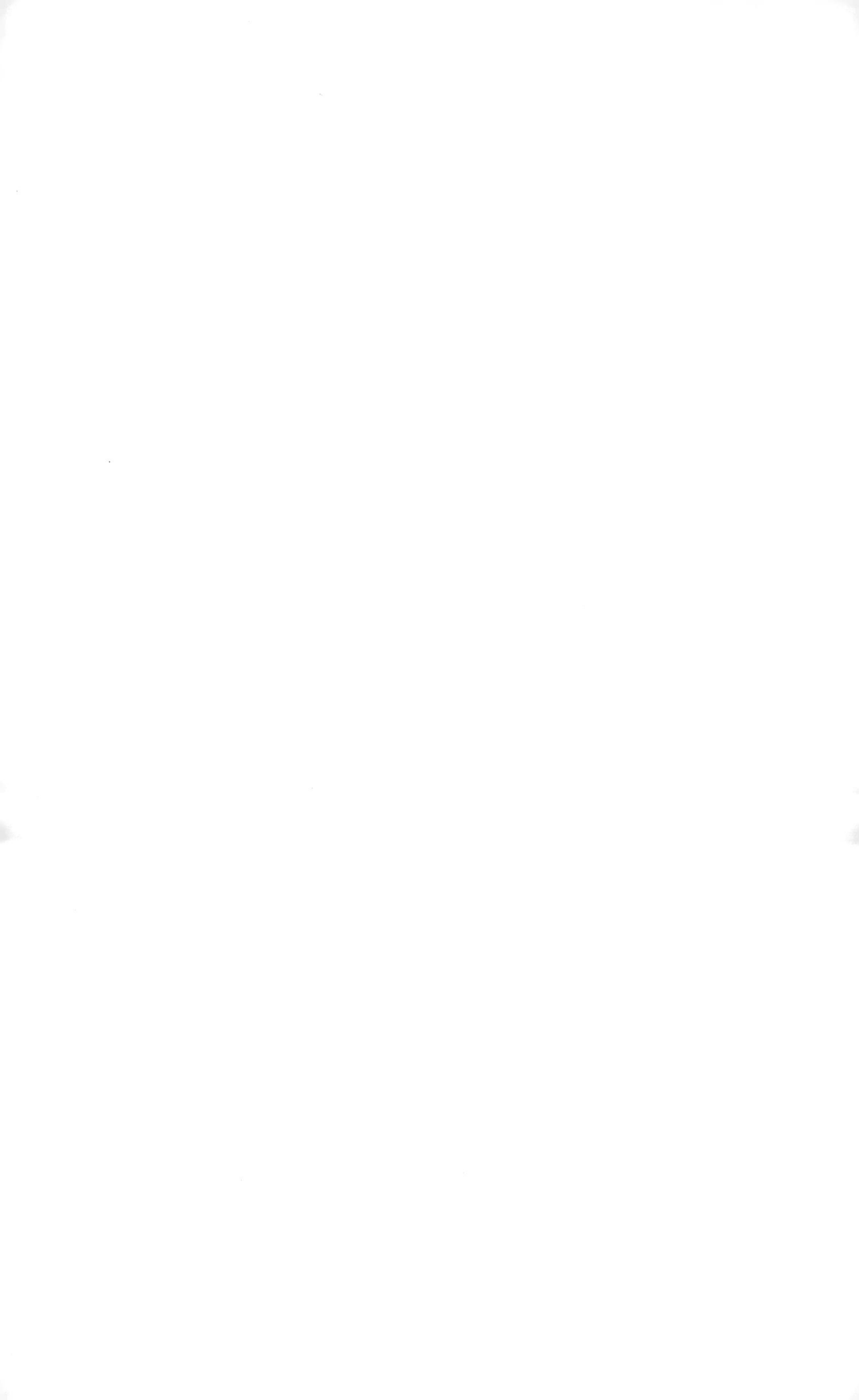

Chapter 3
Materials and Methods

Abstract In this chapter the materials and the methodology used for this study are elaborated. The materials used are listed in the table in materials section, followed by the solution preparations used in this study. The encapsulation, physical and stability determination methodology of the encapsulated lipase are elaborated in early sections. The methodology used in the optimization of the biodiesel production parameters using encapsulated lipase is elaborated in the later sections followed by the lifecycle analysis and economic analysis of biodiesel production.

3.1 Materials

The materials used in this study and their manufacturing details are listed in the Table 3.1.

κ-carrageenan powder 3 % (w/v) was prepared by adding 3 g κ-carrageenan powder in to a beaker containing 100 ml distilled water and stirred using a temperature controlled magnetic stirrer. The mixture in the beaker was heated at 80 °C until κ-carrageenan dissolved completely and cooled down to 45 °C at the time of use. KCl 2 % (w/v) was prepared by adding 2 g KCl to a beaker containing 100 ml distilled water and stirred well to dissolve the KCl completely using a glass rod. Lipase enzyme solution was prepared by adding desired amount of lipase enzyme powder to a test tube containing phosphate buffer (pH7) and mixed well in a vortex machine to dissolve the lipase. p-NPP solution was prepared by adding desired amount of p-NPP to a beaker containing reagent grade ethanol and stirred well using a glass rod to dissolve p-NPP. Bovine serum albumin solution was prepared by adding desired amount of bovine serum albumin to a test tube containing distilled water and mixed well.

Protein analysis reagent A was prepared by adding 50 ml of 2 % sodium carbonate with 50 ml of 0.1 N NaOH solutions (0.4 g in 100 ml distilled water) in a beaker. Protein analysis reagent B was prepared by adding 10 ml of 1.56 % copper sulphate solution with 10 ml of 2.37 % sodium potassium tartarate solution in a beaker. Analytical reagent (C) was prepared by mixing 2 ml of (B) with 100 ml of (A). Folin–Ciocalteau reagent was prepared by diluting 2 N commercial

© The Author(s) 2015

P. Ravindra, K.R. Jegannathan, *Production of biodiesel using lipase encapsulated in κ-carrageenan*, SpringerBriefs in Bioengineering,
DOI 10.1007/978-3-319-10822-3_3

Table 3.1 List of materials and the manufacturers

Name of the materials	Manufacturer Details
κ-carrageenan (Gelcarin GP-911NF)	FMC Biopolymer (USA)
Refines palm oil	Lam soon edible oil (Malaysia)
0.45 Micron filter (PTFE casing)	Whatman (USA)
Lipase PS	Amano Enzymes (Japan)
p-NPP (Nitrophenyl palmitate)	Sigma Chemicals (USA)
Methyl palmitate (HPLC grade)	
Methyl oleate (HPLC grade)	
Methyl stearate (HPLC grade)	
Methyl linoleate (HPLC grade)	
Diolein (HPLC grade)	
Monoolein (HPLC grade)	
Palmitic acid (HPLC grade)	
Oleic acid (HPLC grade)	
Steric acid (HPLC grade)	
Linoleic acid (HPLC grade)	
Bovine serum albumin (HPLC grade)	
Sodium carbonate	Fisher scientific (USA)
KCl	
Methanol (HPLC grade)	
h-hexane (HPLC grade)	
Iso-Propanol (HPLC grade)	
Folin-Ciocalteau reagent	
Methanol	
Ethanol	
Acetone	
n-Heptane	
Phosphate buffer (pH 7)	
SimaPro 7.1	PRé Consultants, Netherlands

Folin- Ciocalteau reagent 2 N to 1 N by adding an equal volume of distilled water in a beaker.

HPLC solvent (Hexane: iso-Propanol) was prepared by adding hexane and isopropanol (HPLC grade) solvents in the ratio of 4:5 (v/v) in a blue cap bottle and mixed well. Known amount of HPLC standards were added to the binary solvent (Hexane and iso- Propanol 4:5 (v/v) in a test tube and mixed well in vortex machine. Biodiesel sample was prepared by withdrawing 0.5 ml of biodiesel sample from the reaction mixture in a vial and centrifuged at 10,000 rpm for 10 min and 0.1 g of the upper layer from the vial was mixed with 10 ml HPLC binary solvent (Hexane and iso- Propanol 4:5 (v/v) in a test tube and further diluted to obtain 100 μg sample per 20 μl solvent.

3.2   Methods

3.2.1   Lipase Encapsulation

Encapsulation of *Burkholderia cepacia* lipase using κ-carrageenan was carried out using coaxial needle by co-extrusion method (Jegannathan et al. 2009) as shown in Fig. 3.1. The inner and outer diameters of the coaxial needle were 0.8 and 1.6 mm in diameter. The lipase enzyme solution (1 g/ml) in the inner needle and κ-carrageenan solution (3 %) in the outer needle were co-extruded at a flow rate of 5 ml/h and 50 ml/h using a syringe pump (Model TE-331) Thermo (Japan). Refined palm oil was used as the continuous phase and the flow rate of continuous phase was maintained at 60 ml/h using a peristaltic pump, Watson and Marlow (England). The continuous phase stream flowed into a stirred beaker containing 2 % KCl solution and stirred using a magnetic stirrer. After the lipase solution in the syringe pump was extruded out completely, the beaker containing the KCl solution and encapsulated lipase was removed out of the magnetic stirrer. The encapsulated lipase in the beaker was allowed to settle in the aqueous KCl phase and the oil phase was removed from the beaker. The encapsulated lipase was filtered using a sieve and washed to remove excess oil and hardened in KCl solution for 24 h at 4 °C. After 24 h the capsules were filtered, dried in room temperature, and used for further studies.

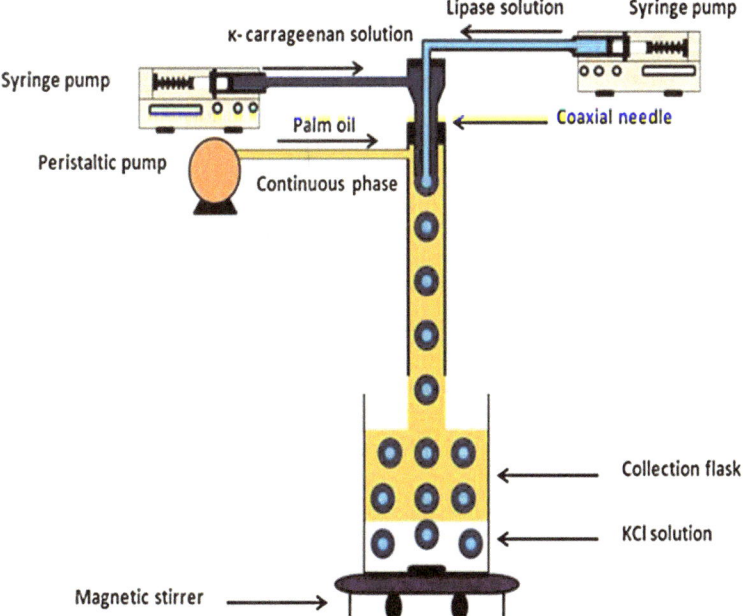

Fig. 3.1 Schematic diagram of encapsulation method (Jegannathan et al. 2009)

In encapsulation, the κ-carrageenan concentration was fixed to 3 % (w/v) due to the thermosensitive characteristic of the κ-carrageenan and enzyme. Clogging in needle could be observed when using κ-carrageenan solution concentration above 3 % (w/v) at 45 °C. Increasing the temperature of encapsulation setup would have favoured to use higher concentration of κ-carrageenan, but the rise in temperature beyond 45 °C may inactivate the enzyme. Thus, the concentration of κ-carrageenan solution was fixed at 3 % (w/v) (Jegannathan et al. 2009).

3.2.2   Capsule Size and Coefficient of Variance

The size and the membrane thickness of the encapsulated *Burkholderia cepacia* lipase in κ-carrageenan produced via co-extrusion technique lipase was measured using the microscopic picture taken by an optical microscope (Eschenbach, USA) attached with a camera (Motic, China) and Motic software. The coefficient of variance of the capsule size was calculated accounting 60 capsules (Jegannathan et al. 2009).

3.2.3   Moisture Content

The moisture content of κ-carrageenan encapsulated *Burkholderia cepacia* lipase was determined by drying a known weight of the encapsulated capsules in a hot air oven at 102 °C until a constant weight was obtained (Jegannathan et al. 2009).

3.2.4   Immobilization Efficiency

The encapsulation efficiency was evaluated in terms of protein coupling (the amount of protein binding to the matrix). The amount of protein content introduced and the amount of protein coupled during immobilization was estimated by Lowry's method using bovine serum albumin as standard. The principle behind the Lowry method of determining protein concentrations is that, the phenol group of tyrosine and trytophan residues (amino acid) in protein will produce a blue purple colour complex, with Folin-Ciocalteau reagent which consists of sodium tungstate molybdate and phosphate. Different dilutions of BSA solutions were prepared by mixing stock BSA solution (100 mg/L) and water in the test tube. From these different dilutions, 1 ml protein solution was pipette out to different test tubes and 2 ml of alkaline copper sulphate reagent (analytical reagent) was added. The solutions were mixed well and incubated at room temperature for 10 min. After incubation, 0.2 ml of reagent Folin Ciocalteau solution (reagent solutions) was added to each tube and incubated for 30 min in dark. The test tube having no BCA solution serves as the blank.

The spectrophotometer was zeroed with blank and the optical density of other samples was measured at 660 nm. The absorbance was plotted against protein concentration to get a standard calibration curve. The absorbance of unknown samples was measured and the concentration of the unknown sample was determined using the standard curve (Jegannathan et al. 2009).

$$\text{Protein coupling yield}\,(\%) = \frac{\text{amount of protein coupled}}{\text{amount of protein   introduced}} \times 100$$

3.2.5   Surface and Internal Morphologies of Encapsulated Lipase

A scanning electron microscope (SEM, Model: JSM-5G1DLV, JEOL, Tokyo, Japan) was used to observe the surface and the internal morphologies of encapsulated lipase capsules. Cross-sectioned samples of κ-carrageenan encapsulated lipase capsules were prepared by cutting the capsules with razor blade for viewing the internal structure using SEM. The Cross-sectioned samples were mounted on metal stubs using double side adhesive tape, dried under vacuum and coated with a platinum layer using a fine coater (JEOL, Japan. Model: JFC-1600). The platinum coated samples were mounted in the samples stub inside the scanning electron microscope and the images were viewed and captured under different angles and magnification.

3.2.6   Interaction Between κ-Carrageenan and Lipase

Interaction of κ-carrageenan and lipase in the capsules were studied using a Fourier transform Infra-red (FTIR) spectroscope (Thermo Fischer, USA. Model: Nicolet 8700). The dried samples of κ-carrageenan powder, lipase powder and κ-carrageenan encapsulated lipase were crushed in a pestle and mortar to fine powder separately and pressed with potassium bromide to pellets in a sample stub. The samples were placed in the sample holder for FTIR analysis. Spectrograms of the samples were collected and analysed for their structural interaction based on their wave number.

3.2.7   Lipase Activity

The activity of free lipase and κ-carrageenan encapsulated *Burkholderia cepacia* lipase were measured by the modified spectrophotometric method of Hung et al. (2003) using p-NPP as substrate. 50 μl of free lipase solution or 100 mg immobilized lipase (*Burkholderia cepacia* lipase encapsulated in κ-carrageenan) was added to 1 ml of 0.05 M phosphate buffer (pH 7) in a test tube. 100 μl of 0.1 %

(w/v) p-NPP was added to the test tube with reaction mixture and placed in incubator maintained at 30 °C. After 5 min of reaction at 30 °C, the reaction was terminated by adding 2 ml of 0.5 N Na_2CO_3. The mixture was centrifuged at 10,000 rpm for 10 min (Centrifuge, Thermo, Germany) and the absorbance of the supernatant was measured at 410 nm using a spectrophotometer, Spectronic (USA). For the blank sample the enzyme solution was added after termination of the reaction. From the measured absorbance, the lipase activity is calculated using the formula

$$\text{Lipase activity} = \left(A_{410nm} / \Delta\varepsilon\right) \times \left(V / \infty\right) \times \left(1/t\right) \times 10^6 \,\mu\text{mole} / \min$$

Where,

A_{410nm} – Absorbance at 410 nm
$\Delta\varepsilon$ – Molar extinction of nitrophenol (15,000 M^{-1} cm^{-1})
V – Total volume of reaction
∞ – Volume of enzyme
t – Reaction time

One unit of activity was defined as the amount of enzyme necessary to hydrolyze 1 μmol p-NPP per min under the conditions of assay.

3.2.8   pH Stability

The pH stability of the free lipase and κ-carrageenan encapsulated *Burkholderia cepacia* lipase was carried out by incubating the immobilized enzyme at 30 °C in the buffers of varying pH in the range of 3–9 for 1 h. After 1 h the capsules were separated from the buffer solution using a filter, dried in room temperature and its catalytic activity was determined as described in lipase activity section. Relative activities were calculated as the ratio of the activity of free lipase and κ-carrageenan encapsulated *Burkholderia cepacia* lipase to the activity at the optimum reaction pH and the results were plotted against pH (Jegannathan et al. 2009).

3.2.9   Temperature Stability

The assessment of thermal stability of the soluble lipase and encapsulated *Burkholderia cepacia* lipase in κ-carrageenan was carried out by incubating the immobilized enzyme at various temperatures in the range of 25–45 °C for 1 h at pH 7 and the capsules were separated from the buffer solution using a filter, dried in room temperature and its catalytic activity was determined as described in activity section. Relative activities were calculated as mentioned in above section and the results were plotted against temperature (Jegannathan et al. 2009).

3.2.10 Solvent Stability

The stability of encapsulated *Burkholderia cepacia* lipase in κ-carrageenan in various solvents including phosphate buffer pH 7, methanol, ethanol, iso-propanol, acetone, n-heptane and n-hexane was studied by incubating the immobilized enzyme at various solvents at 30 °C for 1 h. Thereafter, the capsules were separated from the solvents using a filter, dried in room temperature and the immobilized enzyme was assayed for relative lipase activity. The activity of *Burkholderia cepacia* lipase in κ-carrageenan suspended in phosphate buffer was taken as the reference for calculating relative activity (Jegannathan et al. 2009).

3.2.11 Storage Stability

The κ-carrageenan encapsulated *Burkholderia cepacia* lipase was stored in 27 °C and the activities were measured periodically over duration of 10 days. The activities were expressed as the percentage retention of their activities at various time intervals (Jegannathan et al. 2009).

3.2.12 Reusability of the Immobilized Lipase

To evaluate the reusability of the κ-carrageenan encapsulated *Burkholderia cepacia* lipase, the capsules were washed with buffer solution after use in hydrolysis of p-NPP and suspended again in fresh aliquot of the substrate to measure the enzymatic activity. Relative activities were calculated as mentioned above and plotted against reuse (Jegannathan et al. 2009).

3.2.13 Reaction Conditions and Optimization of the Biodiesel Production in Stirred Tank Batch Reactor

The enzymatic transesterification reactions using encapsulated lipase were carried out in a 50 ml baffled conical flask (Corning, USA) as a stirred tank reactor, in an orbital shaker incubator (Heidolph, Germany). A standard set of reaction conditions were used as the base line in the optimization studies. The initial conditions were 10 g palm oil, 3 g methanol (methanol to oil ratio of 8.2), 0.5 g water, 400 mg free lipase or 3 g immobilized lipase (weight basis), 30 °C, $14.3 \times g$ relative centrifugal force (RCF) and 24 h reaction time. For example, when the effect of oil and methanol ratio was investigated, the remaining reaction conditions were unchanged at: 10 g palm oil, 3 g methanol, 0.5 g water, 3 g immobilized lipase PS, $14.3 \times g$ RCF and 24 reaction time (Jegannathan et al. 2010).

3.2.14   Effect of Oil and Methanol Ratio

Experiments were performed in a stirred tank reactor to optimize the amount of methyl ester production by varying the alcohol concentration. The molar ratio of oil to methanol was varied from 1:1 to 1:12 with other conditions remaining the same as mentioned in the reaction setup and optimization section (Jegannathan et al. 2010).

3.2.15   Effect of Water Concentration

The effect of water concentration in transesterification of palm oil in the range of 0 to 2.0 g and at optimum oil: alcohol molar ratios of methanol with respect to palm oil were examined. Other reaction parameters remaining the same as mentioned in the reaction setup and optimization section (Jegannathan et al. 2010).

3.2.16   Effect of Enzyme Loading

Experiments were performed to determine the effect of enzyme loading on the extent of the transesterification reaction. Immobilized enzyme loading in the range of 0-7 g were examined in the transesterification of palm oil with methanol. One gram of immobilized enzyme corresponds to 80 mg free enzyme (based on mass balance) in these reactions. Other reaction parameters remaining the same as mentioned in the reaction setup and optimization section (Jegannathan et al. 2010).

3.2.17   Effect of Temperature

Experiments were performed to determine the effect of temperature on the extent of the transesterification reaction. The temperature was studied in the range of 20-40 °C. Other reaction parameters remain the same as mentioned in the reaction setup and optimization section (Jegannathan et al. 2010).

3.2.18   Effect of Reaction Time

The effect of reaction time on the transesterification reaction was studied in the reaction time range of 0-78 h. Other reaction parameters remain the same as mentioned in the reaction setup and optimization section (Jegannathan et al. 2010).

3.2.19 Effect of Mixing Intensity

Effect of mixing intensity on the transesterification reaction was studied in the range from 0 to $23.7 \times g$ (RCF). Other reaction parameters remain the same as mentioned in the reaction setup and optimization section (Jegannathan et al. 2010).

3.2.20 Reusability of Immobilized Enzyme

Experiments were performed to examine the recyclability and stability of the immobilized lipase. After each transesterification reaction, lipase – containing capsules were recovered by filtration and subsequently reused. This procedure was repeated several times to examine the extent of the stability of the immobilized enzyme (Jegannathan et al. 2010).

3.2.21 Reaction Conditions and Optimization of Biodiesel Production in Packed Bed Batch Reactor

The enzymatic transesterification reactions were carried out in a double walled column (1 cm dia and 21 cm long) (Corning, USA) as a packed bed reactor attached with a recirculated water bath for temperature control. Transesterification of palm oil with methanol was initiated by circulation of the mixed palm oil/alcohol/water reactants from the reactor substrate reservoir through the packed bed reactor. From the previous studies on stirred tank batch reactor the palm oil -to-alcohol mole ratio of 1:7, palm oil 40 g, 21 g immobilized lipase and 4 g water at 30 °C was used throughout this study.

3.2.22 Effect of Flow Rate

Effect of flow rate on the transesterification reaction in packed bed reactor was studied in the range from 0.5 to 2 ml/min for 24 h reaction time. Other reaction parameters were as stated earlier in the reaction setup and optimization section.

3.2.23 Effect of Reaction Time

Effect of reaction time on the transesterification reaction in packed bed reactor was studied by extending the reaction time to 300 h. Other reaction parameters were as stated earlier in the reaction setup and optimization section.

3.2.24 Biodiesel Sampling and Analysis

The composition of the reaction mixture samples was determined by the modified High Performance Liquid Chromatography (HPLC) method of Holčapek et al. (1999) using a Hitachi 7000 HPLC, equipped with a degasser, a binary pump and auto sampler with a Chromatographic column- Zorbax Eclipse XDB-C18 capillary column (4.6 mm – 250 mm – 5 μm) and UV/VIS detector. Solvent A (Methanol) and solvent B (iso-Propanol/ n-hexane, 5:4 by volume) were used as the mobile phase. The samples of the reaction mixture at different time intervals were centrifuged at 1,677 × g RCF for 10 min, a known amount of the upper layer was dissolved into a mixture of iso-Propanol/ n-hexane, 5:4 v/v and injected using an auto sampler. All the samples and solvents were filtered using 0.45 μm Millipore filter. The flow rate of a binary solvent mixture (Methanol, solvent A, and iso-Propanol/ n-hexane, 5:4 by volume, solvent B) was 1 ml/min with a linear gradient (from 100 % A to 40 % A + 60 % B in 30 min). Column temperature was maintained at a constant value of 40 °C. The components were detected at 205 nm. The fatty acids were identified by comparison of retention times of the oil components with those of standards. The relative HPLC areas and the component mass were calibrated using known standard compositions. The percentage conversion was taken as the conversion of triglycerides to methyl esters, monoglycerides, and diglycerides (Jegannathan et al. 2010).

3.2.25 Life Cycle Assessment (LCA)

The purpose of this study was to compare the environmental impacts of various process of biodiesel production at the industrial scale. These include the use of alkali, soluble enzyme catalysts, and immobilized enzyme catalyst in biodiesel production. It should be borne in mind that, currently, there are no industrial-scale processes for biodiesel based on enzymatic transesterification. An outcome of this study is to identify the scientific and technical barriers to overcome for a biological route to be competitive with established inorganic routes.

3.2.26 Goal and Scope of the Study

The Life Cycle Assessment of palm biodiesel production using soluble enzyme catalyst, immobilized enzyme catalyst and alkali catalyst were compared using SimaPro 7.1 (LCA software) and the impact categories based on Eco-indicator 99 (Assessment tool) to characterize the inventory data. The study encompasses all the processes and their inputs, such as chemicals, energy, the production of the inputs, transportation of the materials, and all the emissions generated. The system boundary used in this study is shown in Fig. 3.2 (Alkali catalyst), Fig. 3.3 (Soluble enzyme

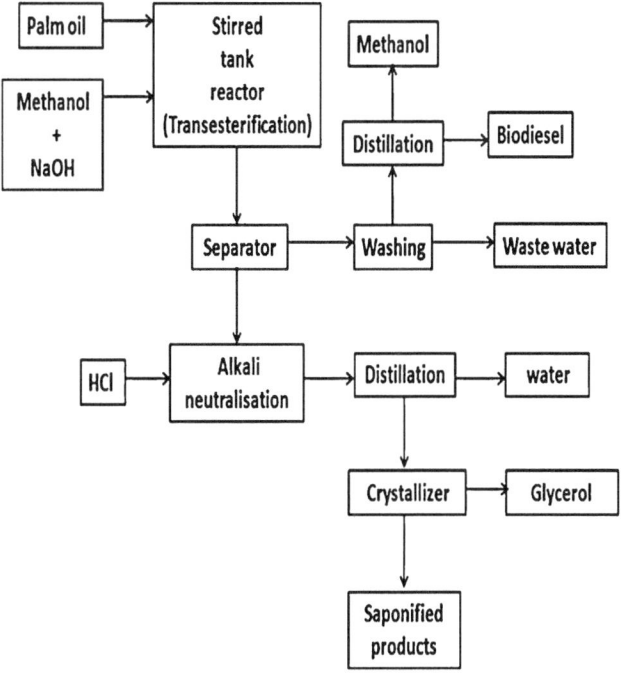

Fig. 3.2 Flow chart of biodiesel production using alkali catalyst (Jegannathan et al. 2011b)

catalyst) and Fig. 3.4 (Immobilized enzyme catalyst). The Process conditions (Table 3.2) for biodiesel production, raw materials and energy requirement data for each method of various capacities is given in Table 3.3 (for alkali catalyst); Table 3.4 (for soluble catalyst) and Table 3.5 (for immobilized enzyme catalyst). After obtaining the materials and energy uses for biodiesel production using alkali catalyst, soluble enzyme catalyst and immobilized catalyst these results were used as inputs for the inventory analysis. The data for lipase production and κ-carrageenan production were adapted from Pooja et al. (2001), Eswaran et al. (2004) and Jegannathan et al. (2009).

3.2.27   Impact Assessment

Environmental impacts of each process considering 11 categories were estimated and the results were reported in percentage and ecopoints (kpt). The 11 categories includes, climate change, carcinogens, respiratory organics, inorganics, ozone layer depletion, ecotoxicity, acidification/ eutrophication, minerals, radiation, land use and fossil fuels.

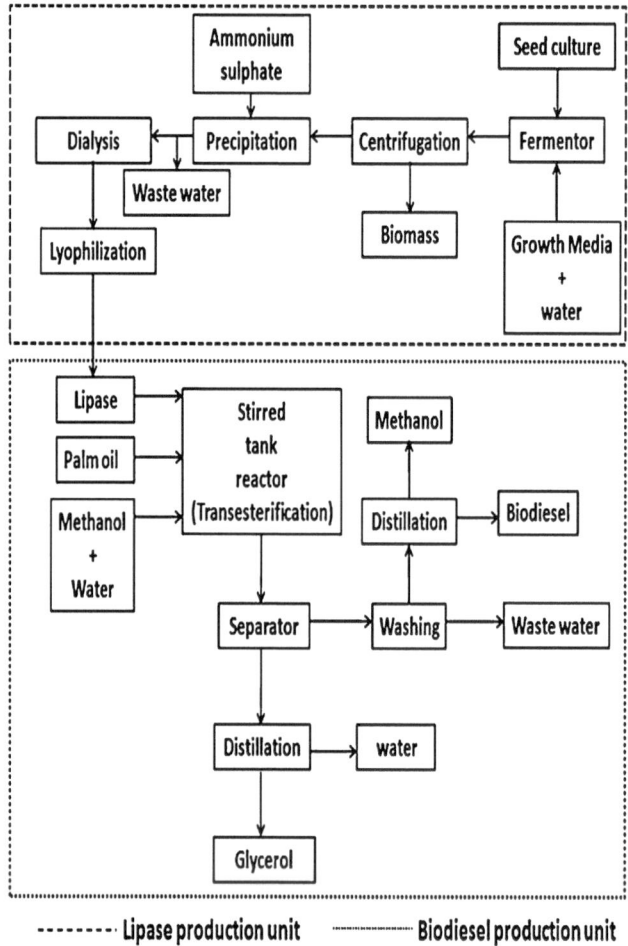

Fig. 3.3 Flow chart of biodiesel production using soluble enzyme catalyst (Jegannathan et al. 2011b)

3.2.28   Inventory Analysis

Table 3.2, Table 3.3, Table 3.4, Table 3.5

3.2.29   Economic Assessment of Biodiesel Production

To assess the biodiesel manufacturing costs, the equipment cost and the plant cost involved in a biodiesel production capacity of 10^3 tonnes/year were estimated by considering the current market cost. Variable costs were calculated on the basis of

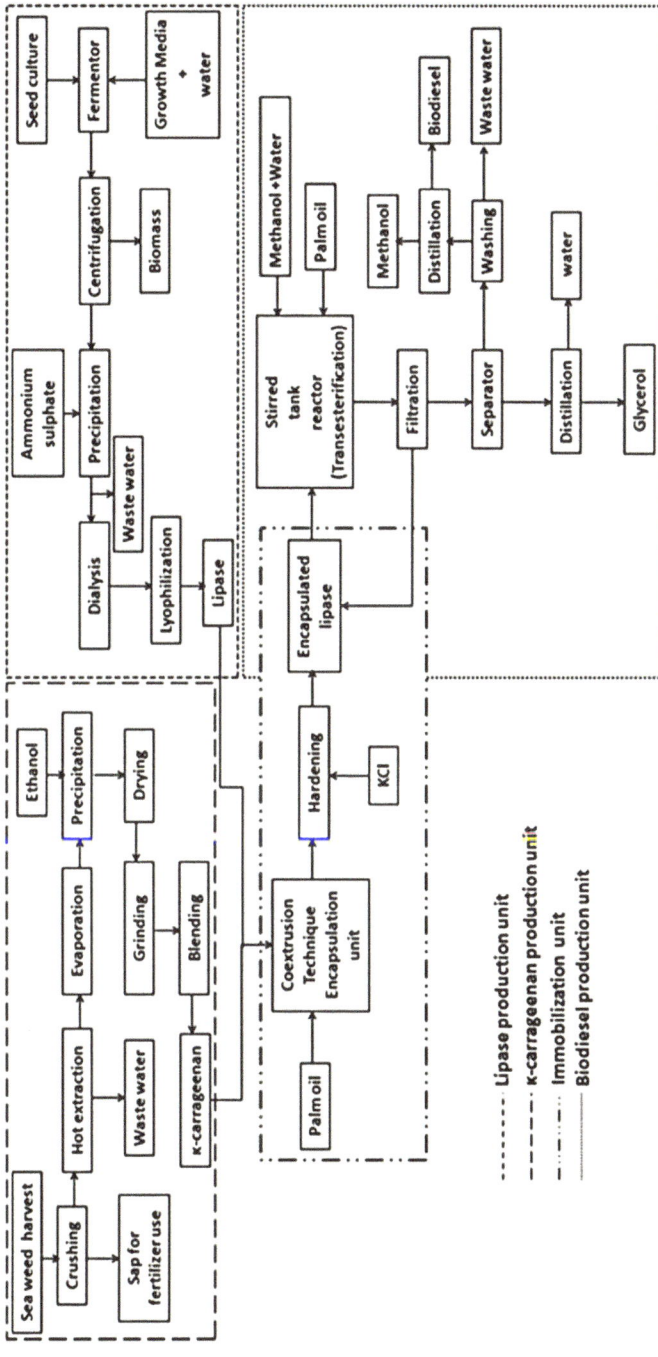

Fig. 3.4 Flow chart of biodiesel production using immobilized enzyme catalyst (Jegannathan et al. 2011b)

Table 3.2 Process conditions for biodiesel production (Jegannathan et al. 2011b)

Raw materials and process parameters	Alkali catalyst	Soluble enzyme	Immobilized enzyme
Oil used	Palm oil	Palm oil	Palm oil
Catalyst used	NaOH	lipase PS	Encapsulated lipase PS
Catalyst fraction	0.1 % of oil (mass)	0.4 % of oil (mass)	50 % of oil (mass)
Alcohol used	Methanol	Methanol	Methanol
Alcohol to oil ratio	7:1	7:1	7:1
Oil conversion	95 %	99 %	99 %
Reactor temperature	60 °C	30 °C	30 °C
Reactor pressure	4 bar	1 bar	1 bar
Reaction time	1.5 h	72 h	72 h

Table 3.3 Materials and energy used to produce biodiesel using alkali catalyst (Jegannathan et al. 2011b)

Production capacity	kg	1,000	5,000	10,000
Materials				
Palm oil	kg	995	4,975	9,950
Methanol	kg	263	1,315	2,630
Sodium hydroxide	kg	10	50	100
Hydrochloric acid	kg	38	190	380
Water	kg	147	735	1,470
Energy				
Electricity	kWh	8.6	43	86
Steam	kg	1,820	9,100	18,200

Table 3.4 Materials and energy used to produce biodiesel using soluble enzyme catalyst (Jegannathan et al. 2011b)

Production capacity	kg	1,000	5,000	10,000
Materials				
Palm oil	kg	1,050	5,250	10,500
Methanol	kg	263	1,315	2,630
Starch from corn	kg	30	150	300
Ammonium sulphate	kg	10	50	100
Magnesium sulphate	kg	1	5	10
Protein from corn	kg	20	100	200
Water	kg	1,200	6,000	12,000
Energy				
Electricity	kWh	20	100	200
Steam	kg	1,540	7,700	15,400

the quantities and the unit prices of raw materials, products, and utilities; fixed costs were calculated on the basis of plant costs and employee costs (Tsutomu et al. 2009). The procedure for estimating the production costs is as follows:

Basic design of biodiesel processes for obtaining a capacity of 1,000 tonnes/year.

- Development of process blocks flow sheets.
- Development of process time charts for achieving a capacity of 1,000 tonnes/year.

Table 3.5 Materials and energy used to produce biodiesel using immobilized enzyme catalyst (Jegannathan et al. 2011b)

Production capacity	kg	1,000	5,000	10,000
Materials				
Palm oil	kg	1,100	5,080	10,055
Methanol	kg	263	1,315	2,630
Water	kg	1,300	2,100	3,000
Ethanol	kg	20	20	20
κ-carrageenan from sea weed	kg	100	100	100
Starch from corn	kg	30	30	30
Magnesium sulphate	kg	1	1	1
Protein from corn	kg	20	20	20
Ammonium sulphate	kg	10	10	10
Energy				
Electricity	kWh	30	100	200
Steam	kg	1,800	5,000	10,000

- Development of material and energy balances for achieving a capacity of 1,000 tonnes/year.
- Development of equipment lists for obtaining a capacity of 1,000 tonnes/year.
- Estimation of equipment costs for obtaining a capacity of 1,000 tonnes/year.
- Estimation of the plant costs for obtaining a capacity of 1,000 tonnes/year.
- Estimation of plant costs for obtaining a capacity ranging from 1,000 tonnes/year.
- Estimation of variable costs for obtaining a capacity of 1,000 tonnes/year.
- Estimation of fixed costs for obtaining capacities ranging from 1,000 tonnes/year.

3.2.30 Process Flow Sheets, Time Chart, and Costs

Three different batch processes were designed to produce biodiesel from refined palm oil. Figure 3.2, Biodiesel production using alkali catalyst process, which is characterized by a homogeneous NaOH catalyst, Fig. 3.3 Biodiesel production using soluble enzyme catalyst process, which is characterized by a homogeneous lipase catalyst, Fig. 3.4, Biodiesel production using immobilized enzyme catalyst process, which is characterized by a heterogeneous lipase catalyst (encapsulated lipase). Process time charts for each process are shown in Figs. 3.5, 3.6 and 3.7. Each process time chart was developed on the basis of a biodiesel production using different processes. Equipment specifications, procurement costs, total plant investment costs, variable costs and fixed costs for the different processes are listed in Table 3.7; Table 3.8. These values were obtained from literature (Tsutomu et al. 2009; You et al. 2008; Sakai et al. 2009) and some data were used from experimentation in this study.

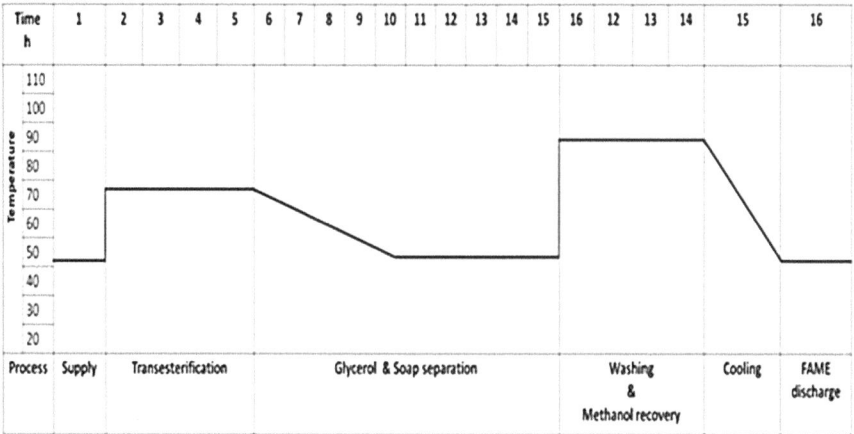

Fig. 3.5 Process time charts for biodiesel production using alkali catalyst (Jegannathan et al. 2011a)

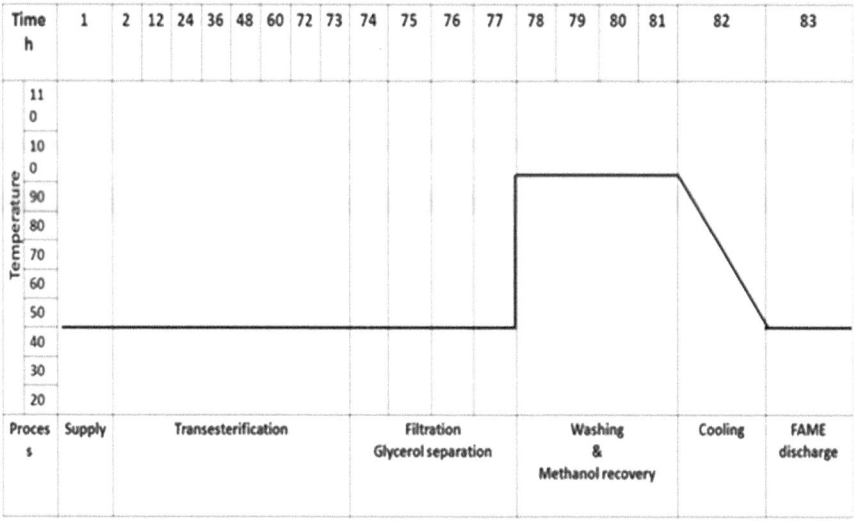

Fig. 3.6 Process time charts for the biodiesel production using soluble enzyme catalyst processes (Jegannathan et al. 2011a)

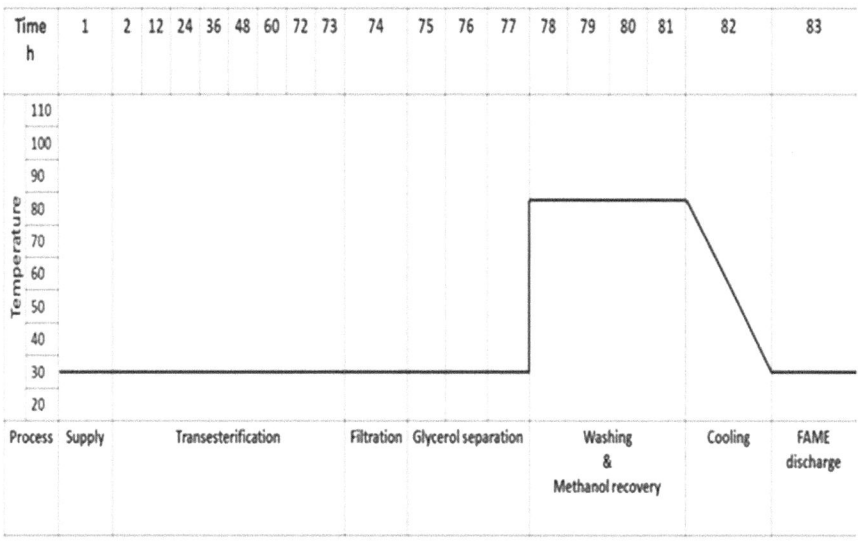

Fig. 3.7 Process time charts for the biodiesel production using immobilized enzyme catalyst (Jegannathan et al. 2011a)

Table 3.6 Equipment specifications and procurement costs for biodiesel production with a capacity of 1,000 tonne using different catalytic processes (Jegannathan et al. 2011a)

		Price $		
Service specification	Capacity	Alkali catalyst process	Soluble enzyme catalyst	Immobilized enzyme catalyst
Palm oil tank	30 kl	27,272	27,272	27,272
Fresh methanol tank	10 kl	27,273	27,273	27,273
Hot water tank	10 kl	12,121	12,121	12,121
FAME tank	6 kl	27,272	27,272	27,272
Waste glycerol tank	2 kl	4,000	4,000	4,000
Waste water tank	2 kl	4,000	4,000	4,000
Oil pump	10 kl/h	3,636	3,636	3,636
Fresh methanol pump	3 kl/h	2,727	2,727	2,727
Hot water pump	3 kl/h	2,727	2,727	2,727
FAME pump	15 kl/h	3,636	3,636	3,636
Waste glycerol pump	10 kl/h	3,182	3,182	3,182
Waste water pump	10 kl/h	3,182	3,182	3,182
NaOH storage unit	2 kl	4,000		
Lipase storage unit	2 kl		4,000	4,000
Encapsulation unit				4,000

(continued)

Table 3.6 (continued)

Service specification	Capacity	Price $		
		Alkali catalyst process	Soluble enzyme catalyst	Immobilized enzyme catalyst
Raw material & product yard total		125,028	125,028	129,028
Transesterification vessel	6 kl	100,364	501,820	501,820
Methanol vessel	1 kl	11,727	11,727	11,727
Waste water vessel	0.2 kl	2,045	2,045	2,045
FAME vessel	4 kl	5,618	5,618	5,618
Waste glycerol vessel	0.5 kl	6,045	3,045	3,045
Waste water vessel	0.5 kl	6,045	3,045	3,045
FAME heater	10 m^2	27,273	27,273	27,273
Vessel condenser	10 m^2	27,273	27,273	27,273
Vessel after cooler	5 m^2	8,182	8,182	8,182
FAME filter(1)	5 m^2	9,091	9,091	9,091
FAME filter(2)	5 m2	9,091	9,091	9,091
FAME pump	10 kl/h	3,182	3,182	3,182
Methanol pump	3 kl/h	2,727	2,727	2,727
FAME pump	10 kl/h	3,182	3,182	3,182
Waste glycerol pump	3 kl/h	2,727	2,727	2,727
Waste water pump	3 kl/h	2,727	2,727	2,727
Main process yard total		227,299	622,755	622,755
Cooling tower	540,000 kJ/h	20,636	13,636	13,636
Cooling water tank	5 kl	9,091	9,091	9,091
Cooling water pump	40 kl/h	2,727	2,727	2,727
Cooling water pump	40 kl/h	2,727	2,727	2,727
Chilling unit	69,000 kJ/h	27,273	27,273	27,273
Chilling water tank	1 kl	4,545	4,545	4,545
Chilling water pump	3 kl/h	2,727	2,727	2,727
Chilling water pump	3 kl/h	2,727	2,727	2,727
Steam boiler unit	500 kg/h	45,455	45,455	45,455
Hot oil heater unit	800 MJ/h	72,727	72,727	72,727
Vacuum pump unit	51 kl/h	9,091	9,091	9,091
Air compressor unit	75 N m^3/h	18,182	18,182	18,182
Nitrogen generator unit	15 N m^3/h	63,636	33,636	33,636
Utility yard total		281,544	244,544	244,544
Equipment cost		633,871	992,327	996,327

Table 3.7 Total plant investment costs for biodiesel production with a capacity of 1,000 tonne using different catalytic processes (Jegannathan et al. 2011a)

Specification	Percentage	Price $ Alkali catalyst process	Soluble enzyme catalyst	Immobilized enzyme catalyst
Equipment	100	633,871	992,327	996,327
Installation	10	63,387.1	99,232.7	99,632.7
Piping	30	190,161.3	297,698.1	298,898.1
Insulation & painting	5	31,693.55	49,616.35	49,816.35
Civil & structure	70	443,709.7	694,628.9	697,428.9
Electric & Instrumentation	35	221,854.9	347,314.5	348,714.5
Computer system	25	158,467.8	248,081.8	249,081.8
Engineering & Supervising	36	228,193.6	357,237.7	358,677.7
General	22	139,451.6	218,311.9	219,191.9
Plant cost		2,110,790	3,304,449	3,317,769

Table 3.8 Variable costs and fixed costs for biodiesel production with a capacity of 1 tonne using different catalytic processes (Jegannathan et al. 2011a)

Expenses	Price ($)	Alkali catalyst Quantity	Cost	Soluble enzyme catalyst Quantity	Cost	Immobilized enzyme catalyst Quantity	Cost
Raw material							
Palm oil	0.56/kg	995	557.2	995	557.2	1,050	588
Methanol	0.45/kg	263	118.35	263	118.35	263	118.35
Tap water	2.27/tonne	147	2.27	130	2.27	130	2.27
Sodium Hydroxide	1.82/kg	10	18.2				
HCl	2/kg	38	76				
lipase	150/kg			40	6,000	8	1,200
κ-carrageenan	10/kg					10	60
KCl	1.8/kg					3	5.4
Utilities							
steam	0.0227/kg	1,820	41.314	1,000	22.7	1,100	24.97
Electricity	0.136/kW h	8.6	1.1696	5	0.68	5	0.68
Man power		8	300	8	300	8	300
Total			1,114.50		7,001.2		2,299.67
By-products							
Glycerol	2/kg	50	100	100	200	100	200
Total	100 %		1,014.50		6,801.2		2,099.67
Depreciation	9 %		91.30		612.10		188.93
Repair	3 %		30.43		204.03		62.99
Interest & Tax	3 %		30.43		204.03		62.99
Total			1,166.67		7,821.37		2,414.63

References

Eswaran K, Ghosh PK, Siddhanta AK, Patolia JS, Periyasamy C, Mehta AS, Mody KH, Ramavat BK, Kamalesh P, Rajyaguru MR, Kulandaivel S, Reddy CRK, Pandya JB, Tewari A (2004) Method for production of carrageenan and liquid fertilizer from fresh seaweeds. US Patent 6,893,479 B2

Holčapek M, Jandera P, Fischer J, Prokes B (1999) Analytical monitoring of the production of biodiesel by high-performance liquid chromatography with various detection methods. J Chromatogr A 858:13–31

Hung TC, Giridhar R, Chiou SH, Wu WT (2003) Binary immobilization of Candida rugosa lipase on chitosan. J Mol Catal B: Enzym 26:69–78

Jegannathan KR, Chan ES, Ravindra P (2009) Physical and stability characteristics of *Burkholderia cepacia* lipase encapsulated in κ-carrageenan. J Mol Catal B: Enzym 58:78–83

Jegannathan KR, Leong JY, Chan ES, Ravindra P (2010) Production of biodiesel from palm oil using liquid core lipase encapsulated in κ-carrageenan. Fuel 89:2272–2277

Jegannathan KR, Chan ES, Ravindra P (2011a) Economic assessment for the production of biodiesel from palm oil using alkali catalysts, soluble enzyme catalysts and immobilized enzyme catalyst. Renew Sustain Energy Rev 15:745–751

Jegannathan KR, Chan ES, Ravindra P (2011b) Life cycle assessment of biodiesel production using alkali, soluble and immobilized enzyme catalyst processes. Biomass Bioenergy 35:4221–4422

Pooja R, Saxena RK, Rani G (2001) A novel alkaline lipase from *Burkholderia cepacia* for detergent formulation. Process Biochem 37:187–192

Sakai T, Kawashima A, Koshikawa T (2009) Economic assessment of batch biodiesel production processes using homogeneous and heterogeneous alkali catalysts. Bioresour Technol 100:3268–3276

Tsutomu S, Ayato K, Tetsuya K (2009) Economic assessment of batch biodiesel production processes using homogeneous and heterogeneous alkali catalysts. Bioresour Technol 100:3268–3276

You YD, Shie JL, Chang CY, Huang SH, Pai CY, Yu YH, Chang CH (2008) Economic cost analysis of biodiesel production: case in soybean oil. Energy Fuels 22:182–189

Chapter 4
Results and Discussion

Abstract κ-carrageenan was used as a matrix for encapsulating lipase PS from *Burkholderia cepacia* and the coextrusion technique was adopted to immobilize lipase. The physicochemical studies showed the diameter of the encapsulated lipase was in the range of 1.3–1.8 mm with an average membrane thickness of 200 μm. The encapsulation efficiency was found to be 42.6 %. The optimum stability was observed at pH 7 and at temperature 40 °C. The Immobilized lipase retained 72.3 % of its original activity after using it for 5 cycles of reuse in hydrolysis of ρ-NPP. The optimum conditions palm oil biodiesel production using encapsulated lipase in a stirred tank immobilized bioreactor (STIBR) were 30 °C, 72 h reaction time and 23.7×g relative centrifugal force. Similarly, the optimal conditions for processing palm oil in a PBBR were 1.5 ml/min and 264 h reaction time. STIBR showed conversion of up to 100 % and the PBR has shown conversion up to 82 %. The kinetic parameters K_m and V_{max} were evaluated for STIBR found to be 600 mol.m^{-3} and 0.84 mol.m^{-3} min^{-1} respectively. The kinetic parameter values were substituted into Michaelis–Menten empirical equation to predict the reaction time. The encapsulated lipase retained 82 % relative conversion after 5 cycles of reuse. The economic assessment of biodiesel production using immobilized enzyme catalyst process was found to be challenging compared to the current alkali process. The Life Cycle Analysis (LCA) studies showed that biodiesel production using immobilized enzyme catalyst has lesser impact on the environment compared to the alkali catalyst and soluble enzyme catalyst. Based on the experimentation and the results, it is concluded that biodiesel production using encapsulated lipase in an immobilized bioreactor open new vistas for the scale up studies of this technology in near future.

4.1 Lipase Encapsulation

Lipase PS from *Burkholderia cepacia* was immobilized by encapsulating lipase in κ-carrageenan via co-extrusion technique. In Literature, encapsulation of lipase in various matrix via co-extrusion technique has been reported (Brandenberger and Widmer 1997; Toreki et al. 2004). However, there is no literature available on lipase encapsulation in κ-carrageenan matrix.

© The Author(s) 2015
P. Ravindra, K.R. Jegannathan, *Production of biodiesel using lipase encapsulated in κ-carrageenan*, SpringerBriefs in Bioengineering,
DOI 10.1007/978-3-319-10822-3_4

4.2 Physical Characteristics of Encapsulated Lipase Capsule

Physical characteristics like size shape and morphology of immobilized enzyme plays a major role in the production process. The size and shape of the immobilized enzyme is crucial for easy handling and reuse of enzyme. Whereas, the morphology shows an insight of the enzyme placement and the pore assembly in the matrix (Cao 2005).

4.2.1 Capsule Size

The microscopic picture of encapsulated lipase produced by coextrusion technique is shown in Fig. 4.1. The encapsulated lipases are spherical in shape with a distinct bilayer showing the inner core of lipase solution and the outer core of κ-carrageenan gel. The diameter range of the encapsulated lipase was found to be 1.3–1.8 mm and

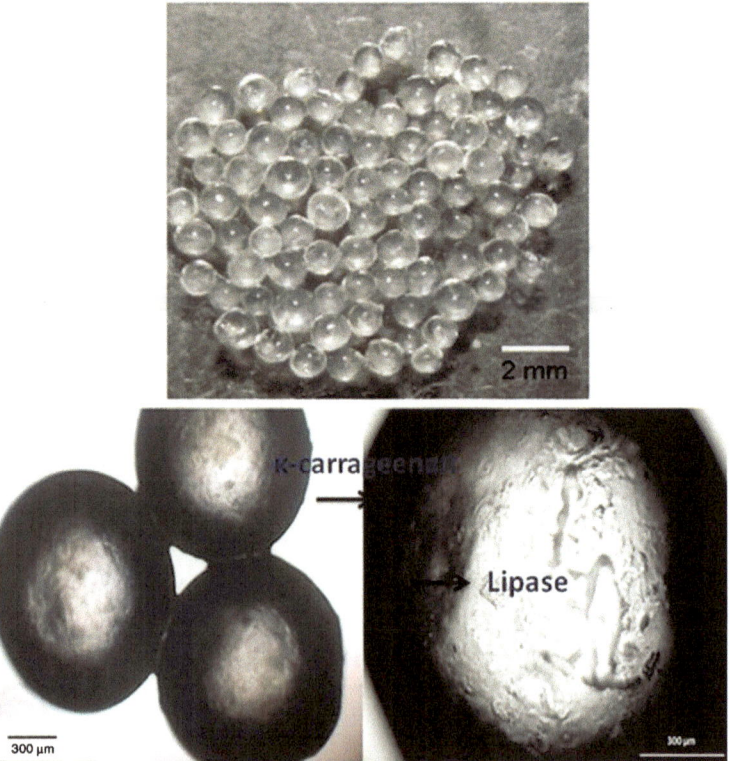

Fig. 4.1 Microscopic pictures of encapsulated lipase showing the liquid core lipase enzyme in the middle surrounded by κ-carrageenan matrix (Jegannathan et al. 2009)

an average membrane thickness of 200 µm. The coefficient of variance accounting 60 capsules was found to be 5 %, indicating that capsules with consistent size were produced. Capsules diameter below this range could be produced by adjusting the encapsulation process parameters but handling those smaller capsules for conducting experiments is tedious. On the other hand, capsules diameter above this range would lead to diffusion problems. In literature, immobilized lipase enzyme in size range of (100 nm–5 mm) produced via different immobilization methods have been reported (Tosa et al. 1979; Betigeri and Neau 2002; Sankalia et al. 2006; Macario et al. 2009) and a size range of 500 µm–5 mm (Orcaire et al. 2006; De queiroz et al. 2006) have been reported produced via encapsulation method.

4.2.2   Moisture Content

The moisture content in the encapsulated lipase was found to be 97 % (Table 4.1). The moisture content of the encapsulated lipase could be further decreased by drying the capsules but this may lead to shrinkage of the κ-carrageenan gel matrix and rupture the encapsulated lipase. Hence, the moisture content was maintained at 97 % throughout the study. In the literature, moisture content of 96.5 % has been reported for lipase immobilized in chitosan via entrapment (Betigeri and Neau 2002) and 48 % in epoxy via covalent immobilization method (Bayramoğlu et al. 2005).

4.2.3   Immobilization Efficiency

The immobilization efficiency was determined in terms of protein coupling. From the data in Table 4.2, the immobilization efficiency was found to be 42.6 %. The immobilization efficiency study shows that there was loss of enzyme and this loss could possibly be due to the agitation in the collection flask containing KCl solution. This was confirmed by the protein assay performed on the aqueous phase (KCl solution). But, the agitation in the collection flask is necessary to keep the capsules

Table 4.1   Moisture content of encapsulated lipase

Weight of encapsulated lipase (initial) (g)	Weight of encapsulated lipase after drying (final) (g)	Moisture content (%)
1	0.03	97

Table 4.2   Immobilization efficiency of the encapsulated lipase (Jegannathan et al. 2009)

Amount of protein introduced (mg/ κ-carrageenan)	Amount of protein coupled (mg/ κ-carrageenan)	Protein coupling Yield (%)
3.52	1.50	42.6

separated in the oil until it is settled in the aqueous phase. If it is not agitated, the capsules tend to diffuse from each other in the oil phase leading to rupture. The immobilization efficiency of various methods have been reported by several investigators and it varies from 30 % to 95 % (Macario et al. 2009; Kılınç et al. 2006; Dizge et al. 2008; Yagiz et al. 2007). The immobilization efficiency can be increased by using a hybrid matrix (κ-carrageenan crosslinked with glutaralde-hyde). However, using glutaraldehyde may cause environmental concerns while disposing the used enzyme.

4.2.4   Surface and Internal Morphologies of Encapsulated Lipase

The scanning electron microscope images were used to show the surface and inter-nal morphologies of encapsulated lipase. Figure 4.2 a–d shows a core-shell struc-ture with lipase surrounded by κ-carrageenan matrix; with a high internal surface area (Fig. 4.2a). Whereas, Fig. 4.2e, f shows the surface morphology of κ-carrageenan matrix with irregular pores in various dimensions. The morphology of the κ-carrageenan encapsulated lipase in its natural gel form could not be shown due to the limitation of scanning electron microscope that only dried samples can be anal-ysed. However, in this study even in the dried condition, a cluster of lipase enzyme particles can be seen in the inner core of capsule (Fig. 4.2). This shows that the lipase has been confined in the middle surrounded by a membrane of κ-carrageenan matrix forming a capsule with bilayer. Similar scanning electron micrographs show-ing the morphology of immobilized lipase prepared via various immobilization methods have been reported (Dizge et al. 2009; Macario et al. 2009; Betigeri and Neau 2002; Tang et al. 2007; Bayramoğlu et al. 2005) in the literature.

4.2.5   Interaction Between κ-Carrageenan and Lipase

FTIR spectra of κ-carrageenan matrix, lipase PS and encapsulated lipase are shown in Fig. 4.3. It is observed, both the free lipases and encapsulated lipase spectrograms showed a typical spectrum of the proteins, with the absorption bands associated with amide group (CONH). Among the wave number range from 1,600 to 1,700 cm-1, it was the amide band, due to the double bond CO stretching, the CN stretching and NH bending. It is also found that the typical bands of D-galactose-4-sulfate, 3,6-anhydro-D-galactose, and ester sulfate stretching in κ-carrageenan and encapsu-lated lipase spectrogram at 844, 949, and 1,276 cm^{-1}. The absence of drastic changes in the spectrogram confirms that there was no strong interaction between the κ-carrageenan matrix and lipase. This could be because of encapsulation

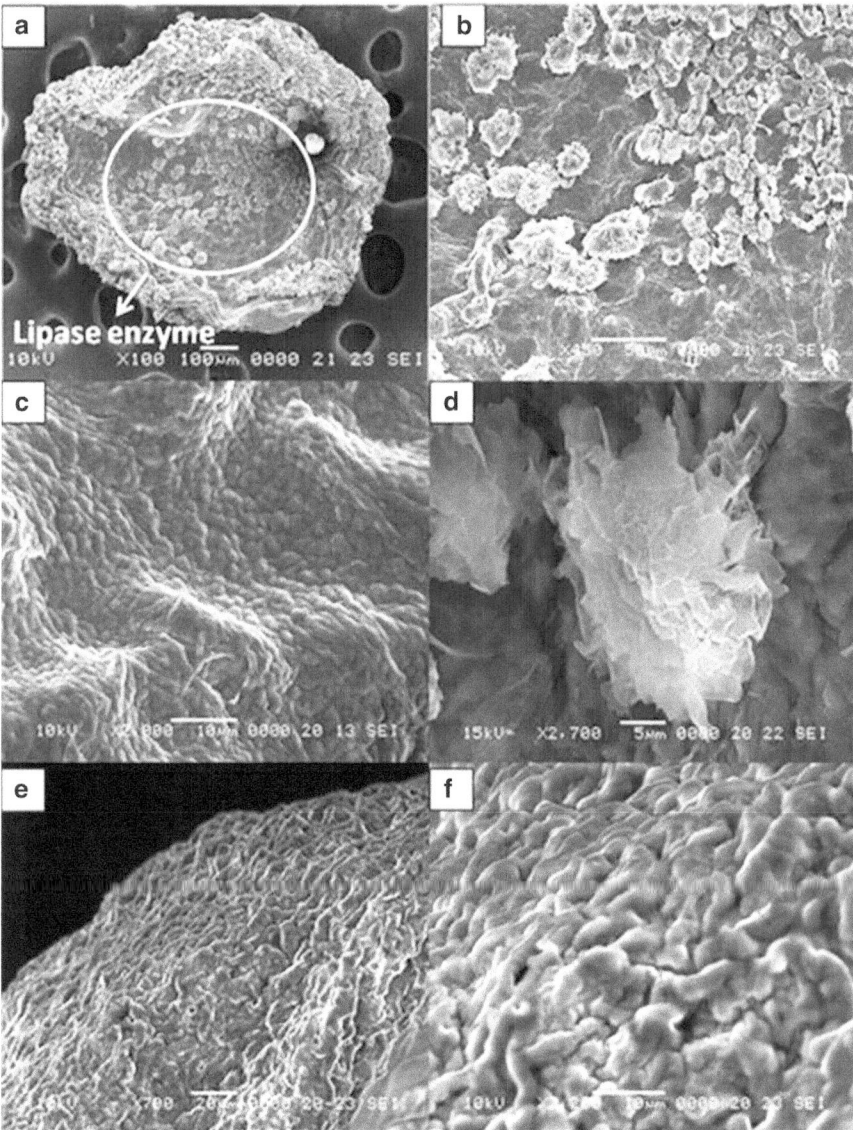

Fig. 4.2 SEM pictures of lipase encapsulated in κ-carrageenan matrix. (**a**) Cross sectional view of encapsulated lipase. (**b**) Lipase surrounded by κ-carrageenan matrix. (**c**) Lipase attached to κ-carrageenan matrix.(**d**) Lipase at higher magnification. (**e**) κ-carrageenan matrix (Outer Layer). (**f**) κ-carrageenan matrix at higher magnification (Outer Layer)

method, where only physical confinement takes place and there was no chemical modification, neither to the matrix nor to the enzyme. FTIR spectra results showing the interaction between various matrix and lipase have been reported in the literature (Chen et al. 2008; Sankalia et al. 2006; Zhang et al. 2005).

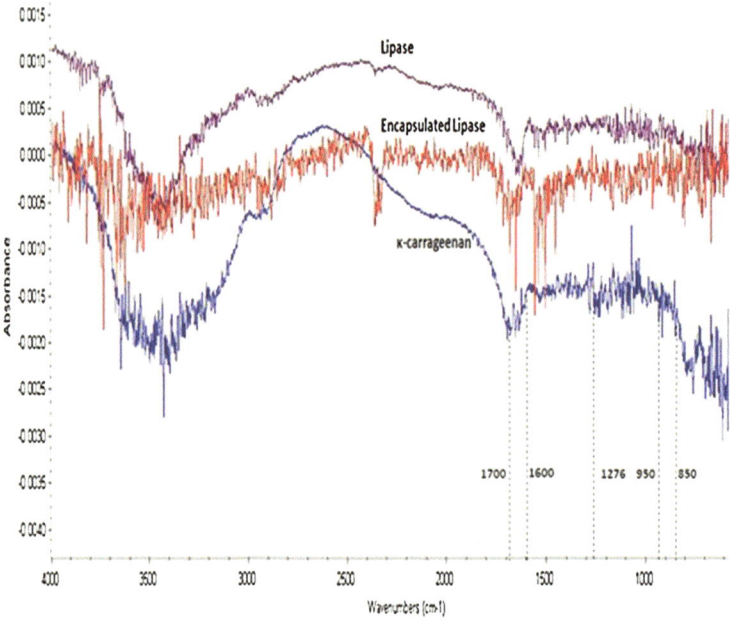

Fig. 4.3 FTIR spectrum of κ-carrageenan, encapsulated lipase and Lipase

4.3   Stability Characteristics of Encapsulated Lipase

It is important to maintain several parameters in production process. Stability of immobilized enzymes as a catalyst in various process parameters is one of the crucial factors. Therefore, the stability of immobilized enzymes were studied with respect to pH, temperature, solvent and storage, and the results are presented in the following sections.

4.3.1   pH Stability

Figure 4.4 shows the relative activity of free lipase and encapsulated lipase as a function of pH. The results revealed that both free lipase and the encapsulated lipase were stable at pH 7. At lower pH the stability of free lipase decreased drastically compared to the immobilized lipase. The possible reason for this could be that the κ-carrageenan matrix protects the enzyme from faster deactivation at lower pH (Jegannathan et al. 2009). Similar results have been reported on pH stability study of immobilized lipases (Dizge et al. 2008; Munjal and Sawhney 2002).

The acid and base dissociation constants were found using Fig. 4.5 and is presented in the Table 4.3. There was no large difference in the dissociation constants of the free lipase and the immobilized lipase indicating that the immobilization method did not alter the structure of the enzyme.

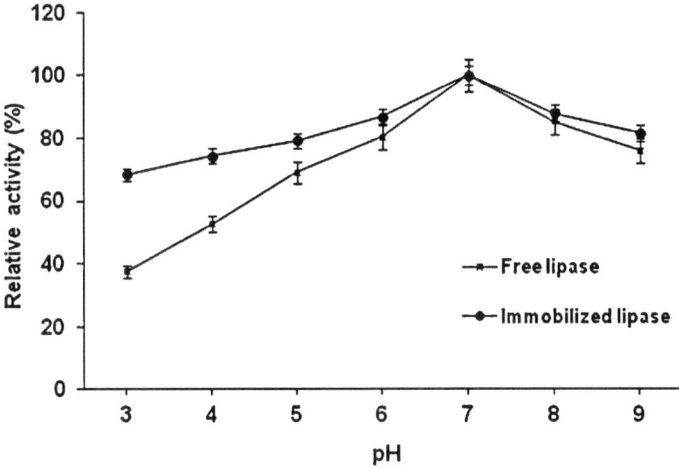

Fig. 4.4   pH stability of free and immobilized lipase at 30 °C (Jegannathan et al. 2009)

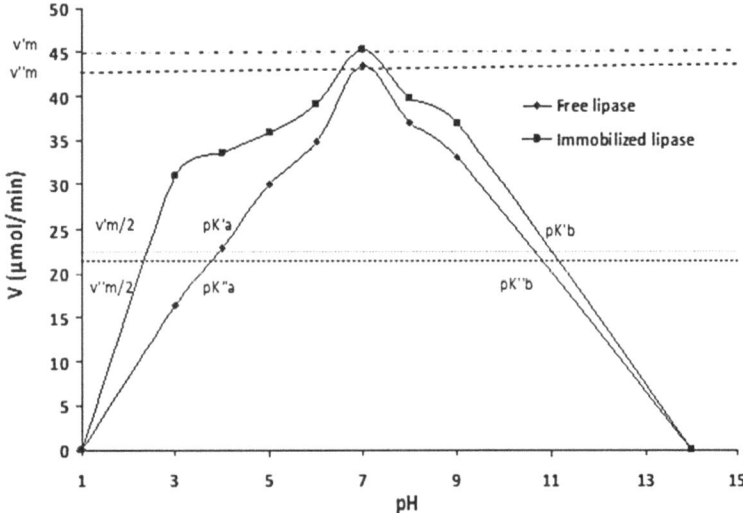

Fig. 4.5   Determination of pK_a and pK_b of free and immobilized lipase at 30 °C

		Immobilized
Dissociation constants	Free lipase	lipase
pKa (acid)	3.8 (pK′a)	2.4 (pK″a)
pKb (base)	11 (pK′b)	11.2 (pK″b)

Table 4.3   Acid and base dissociation constants of free and immobilized lipase

4.3.2 Temperature Stability

Relative catalytic activity as a function of temperature is shown in (Fig. 4.6). The Optimum temperature for free and encapsulated lipase in κ-carrageenan was found to at 40 °C. Encapsulation is the physical enclosure of enzyme within a polymeric membrane. In this method, enzymes do not chemically bond to polymeric matrices. So, the three dimensional structure of the enzymes may not be affected by the immobilization procedure and thus, the optimum temperature stability of the immobilized enzyme was observed similar to free enzyme (Tumturk et al. 2007). On the other hand, the optimal activity of encapsulated lipase could be an advantage of using this catalyst at milder temperature condition favouring low cost production and the environmental impact.

A quantitative evaluation of the temperature effect by calculating the activation energy of the reaction of thermal inactivation was done by plotting the logarithm of the velocity constant V versus the reciprocal of the absolute temperature (Fig. 4.7).

$$V = V_o \, e^{\,E/RT}$$

$$lnV = \ln V_o - E/RT$$

Where

V = Reaction rate constant or velocity constant
V_o = Frequency factor or pre-exponential factor
E = Activation energy, J/mol
R = Gas constant (8.314 J/mol °K)

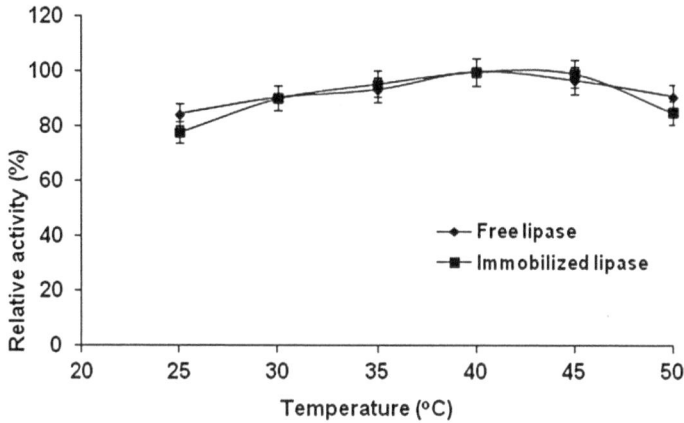

Fig. 4.6 Temperature stability of free and immobilized lipase at pH 7 (Jegannathan et al. 2009)

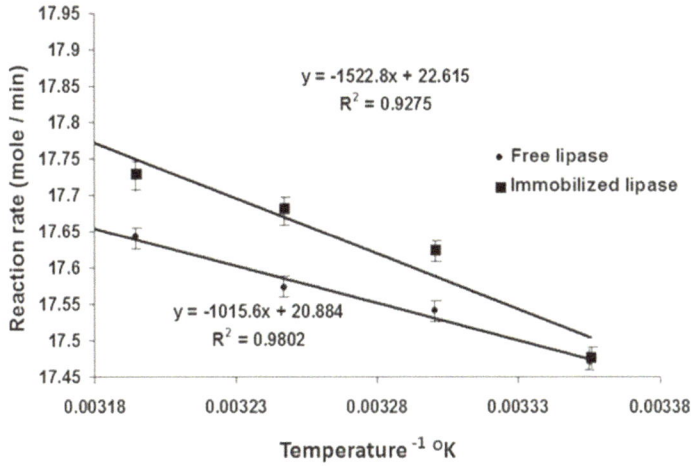

Fig. 4.7 Reaction rate and temperature dependence (Jegannathan et al. 2009)

From Fig. 4.7, the activation energy values of free and immobilized lipase were found to be 122.15 J/mole and 183.16 J/mole, respectively. The high value of activation energy of immobilized lipase confirmed the high sensitivity of reaction towards temperature compared to free lipase. On the other hand the activation energy of free and immobilized lipase 7.8 and 1.25 kJ/mol respectively has been reported by the Vrushali et al. (2009). The lower activation energy of immobilized lipase in comparison to free lipase suggests a change in conformation of the enzyme leading to a requirement for lower energy (Vrushali et al. 2009).

4.3.3   Solvent Stability

The stability of encapsulated lipase in κ-carrageenan in various solvents is shown in (Table 4.4). The activity studies showed that the encapsulated *Burkholderia cepacia* lipase was more stable in alcohol and hexane compared to acetone. *Burkholderia cepacia* lipase showed good stability towards methanol. The high resistance of *Burkholderia cepacia* lipase towards methanol could be an advantage of using this encapsulated lipase in non-aqueous reactions. Similar results were reported in the literature (Kaieda et al. 2001; Shah and Gupta 2006) on solvent stability.

Table 4.4 Solvent stability
of encapsulated lipase
(Jegannathan et al. 2009)

Solvent	Activity (U/100 mg)	Relative activity (%)
Phosphate buffer pH 7	45.1	100
Methanol	42.2	93.5
n-Hexane	39.2	86.9
Ethanol	39.2	86.9
iso-Propanol	36.5	80.9
n-Heptane	31.2	69.1
Acetone	19.7	43.7

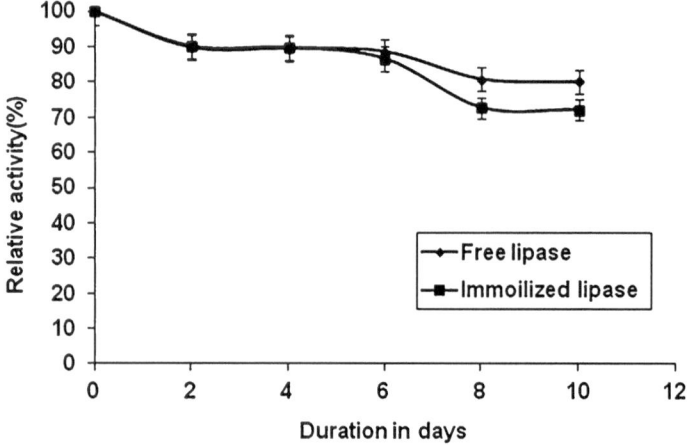

Fig. 4.8   Storage stability of free and immobilized lipase at 27 °C (Jegannathan et al. 2009)

4.3.4   Storage Stability

The encapsulated lipase stored at 27 °C was stable for 10 days, later it disintegrated (Fig. 4.8) indicating that the immobilized lipase could be stored only for limited period. This could be a disadvantage of using natural polymer as a matrix for immobilization. However, in industries the storage problem can be eliminated by storing the encapsulated lipase in appropriate buffer or by having an in-situ encapsulation unit. On the other hand, the disintegration property of κ-carrageenan would be an advantage for safe disposal of the catalyst after use. Similar results have been reported in literature corresponding to the storage stability of immobilized lipase in biopolymers (Hung et al. 2003; Tang et al. 2007)

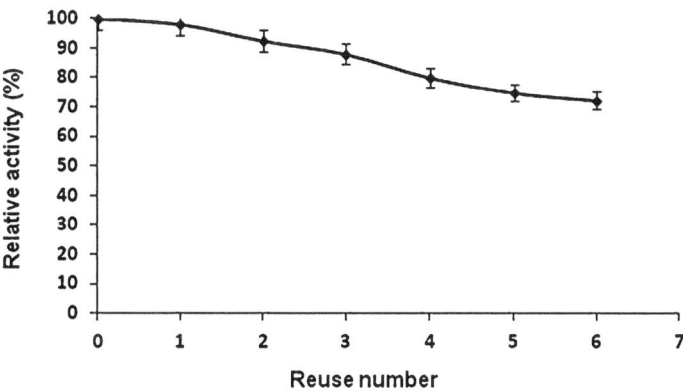

Fig. 4.9 Reuse stability of the immobilized lipase in p- NPP hydrolysis (Jegannathan et al. 2009)

4.3.5   Reusability of Immobilized Lipase

The reusable studies of the encapsulated lipase (Fig. 4.9) showed that the immobilized enzyme retains 72.3 % of its original activity after 6th reuse in the hydrolysis of p-NPP. The leakage of enzyme could be the reason for lower activity of the encapsulated lipase upon reuse. Similar trend has been reported (Tumturk et al. 2007; Soumanou and Bornscheuer 2003) on reusability of immobilized lipase.

4.4   Kinetic Parameters

The effect of substrate concentration on the reaction rate catalyzed by free and immobilized lipase was studied by using Lineweaver-Burk plot, Eadie-Hofstee Plot and Hanes-Woolf plot (Figs. 4.10, 4.11, and 4.12). The kinetic parameters are given in (Table 4.5). A higher K'_m value (K'_m is a measure of affinity of enzyme to substrate) and lower K_{cat} (turn over number) was observed for encapsulated lipase compared to the free lipase. This could be due to lower accessibility of the substrate to the active site by diffusion limitation. The diffusion limitations in the encapsulated lipase could be a disadvantage and similar problems have been reported in the literature. However, mixing the reactor would eliminate diffusion limitations (Pencreac'h et al. 1997; Schuler and Kargi 1992; Anita et al. 1997).

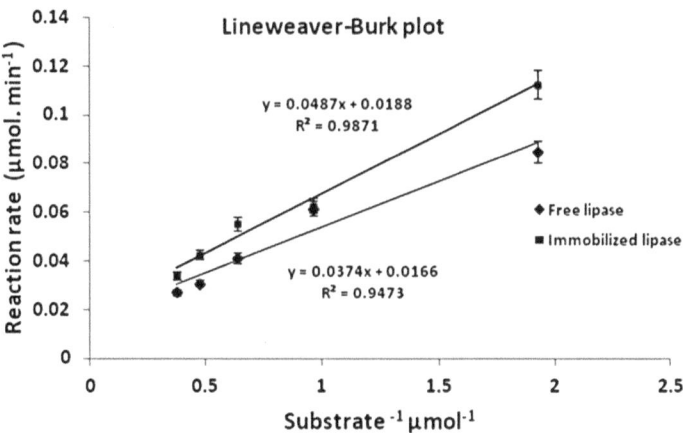

Fig. 4.10 Lineweaver–Burk plot for p- NPP hydrolysis of free and immobilized lipase

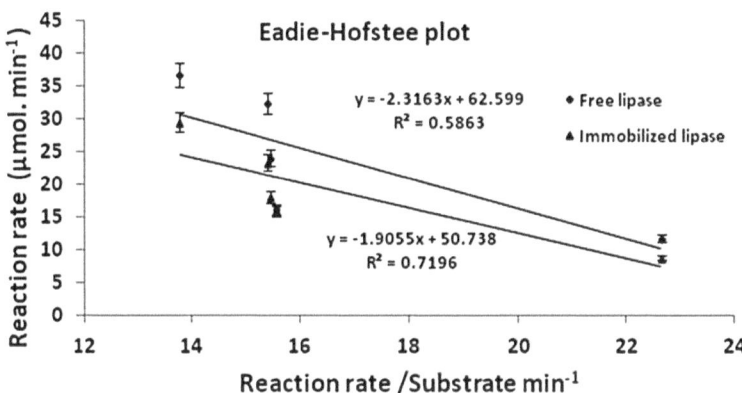

Fig. 4.11 Eadie-Hoftee plot for p- NPP hydrolysis of free and immobilized lipase

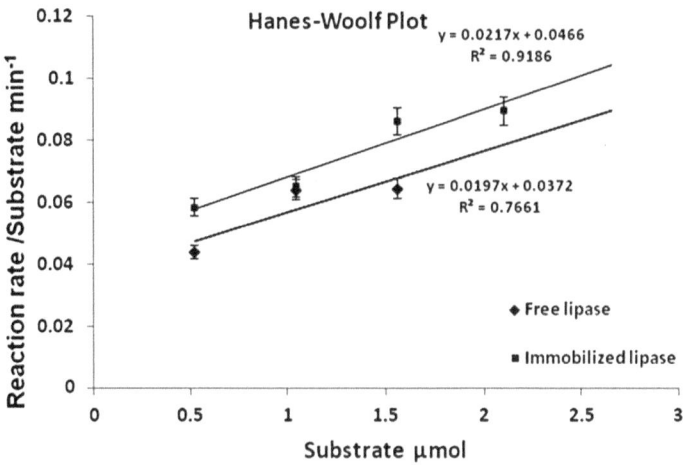

Fig. 4.12 Hanes- Woolf plot for p- NPP hydrolysis of free and immobilized lipase

Table 4.5 Kinetic parameters of free and encapsulated lipase

Parameter	Lineweaver-Burk plot		Eadie-Hofstee plot		Hanes-Woolf plot	
	Free lipase	Immobilized Lipase	Free lipase	Immobilized Lipase	Free lipase	Immobilized Lipase
V'_{max} (µmole/min)	60.24	53.19	62.59	50.73	50.75	46.08
E_0 (µmole)	0.68	0.68	0.68	0.68	0.68	0.68
K'_m (µmole)	2.25	2.59	1.9	2.31	1.87	2.14
K_{cat} min^{-1}	88.58	78.22	92.04	74.60	74.36	67.76

4.5   Biodiesel Production from Palm oil Using Encapsulated Lipase in Batch Immobilized Bioreactor

In the production of biodiesel using immobilized lipase, the process parameters have shown significant contributions towards maximum biodiesel conversion. Hence, the optimization of process parameters have been reported in most of the biodiesel production studies (Salis et al. 2005; Dizge et al. 2009; Zeng et al. 2009). The process parameters for biodiesel production using encapsulated lipase include oil, methanol ratio, water content, reaction temperature, immobilized enzyme loading, reaction time and mixing intensity of the reactor. The effect of these process parameters is presented in the following sections.

4.5.1   Effect of Oil and Methanol Ratio

Effect of alcohol concentration on immobilized lipase shown in (Fig. 4.13) indicated that, an increase in the number of moles of methanol resulted in an increase in methyl ester production. There was no significant increase in methyl ester formation with the increase of molar ratio of oil to methanol beyond 1:7. On the other hand, the higher amount of methanol above stoichiometry level used for the transesterification of palm oil did not inactivate the lipase as reported by (Noureddini et al. 2005; Shah and Gupta 2006; Kaieda et al. 2001).

The high tolerance of *Burkholderia cepacia* lipase towards methanol could be the reason for this behaviour and hence there was no adverse effect by methanol. The reason for high tolerance of *Burkholderia cepacia* lipase towards methanol is due to their conformational change in their protein structure. This could be a major advantage of using *Burkholderia cepacia* lipase in biodiesel production compared to lipase from other sources which gets poisoned at higher methanol content (Watanabe et al. 2001; Samukawa et al. 2000; Du et al. 2005; Lu et al. 2007).

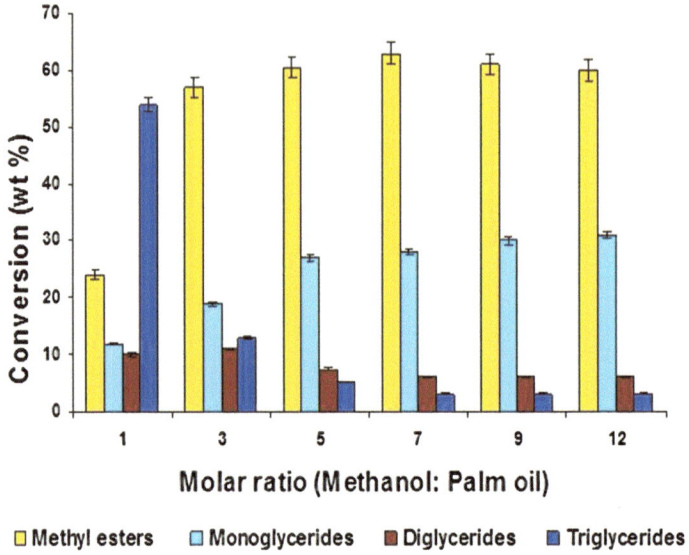

Fig. 4.13 Effect of alcohol concentration on immobilized lipase catalyzed transesterification of palm oil (Process conditions: 5.25 g of immobilized lipase, 10 g of oil, 0.5 g water, a stirring rate of $14.3 \times$ g RCF and a 24 h reaction at 30 °C) (Jegannathan et al. 2010)

4.5.2   Effect of Water Concentration

Results presented in Fig. 4.14 indicate a low enzyme activity at low water concentrations, these observations support that a minimum amount of water is required to activate the enzyme. With the increased addition of water, there was a considerable increase in the methyl esters production showing the enhancement in the activity of the enzyme. The methyl esters formation reached a maximum of about 70 % at 1.0 g water. The increase in the activity of transesterifaction of lipase upon addition of water has been reported previously (Iso et al. 2001; Mittelbach 1990; Li et al. 2006; Yang et al. 2006; Noureddini et al. 2005).

4.5.3   Effect of Immobilized Enzyme Loading

The effect of immobilized enzyme loading in methyl esters formation is shown in Fig. 4.15. The formation of methyl esters was significantly higher for the immobilized enzymes loading of 5.25 g compared with the 1.75 g. At 5.25 g immobilized enzyme loading, the concentration of triglycerides and diglycerides reached negligible levels, while, the formation of monoglycerides and methyl esters were 68 % and 26 % respectively. This result was found to be in accordance with the various reports in literature (Hsu et al. 2001; Shah and Gupta 2006; Kumari et al. 2007; Yagiz et al. 2007).

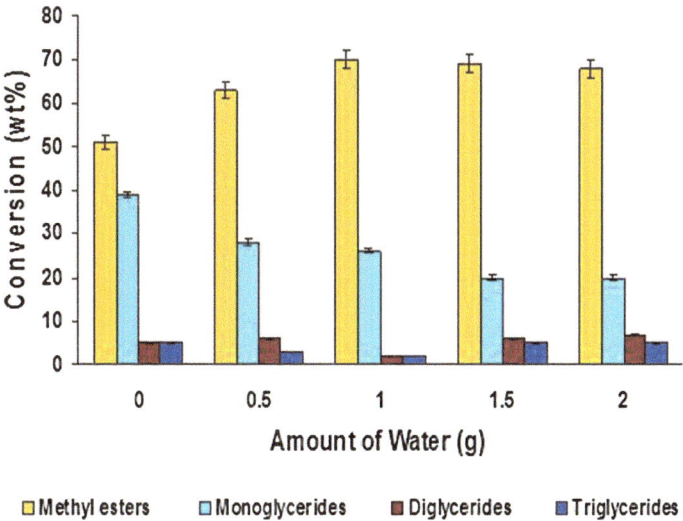

Fig. 4.14 Effect of water concentration on immobilized lipase catalyzed transesterification of palm oil (Process conditions: 5.25 g of immobilized lipase, 10 g of oil, 2.5 g of methanol a stirring rate of 14.3 × g RCF and a 24 h reaction at 30 °C) (Jegannathan et al. 2010)

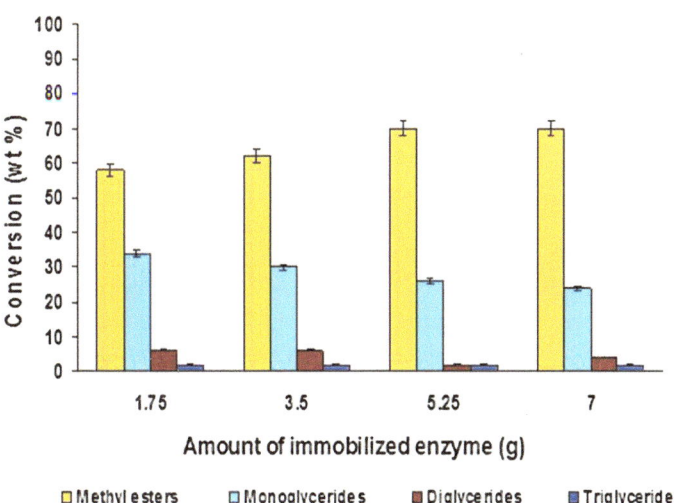

Fig. 4.15 Effect of immobilized enzyme amount transesterification of palm oil (Process conditions: 10 g of oil, 2.5 g of methanol, 1 g of water a stirring rate of 14.3 × g RCF and a 24 h reaction at 30 °C) (Jegannathan et al. 2010)

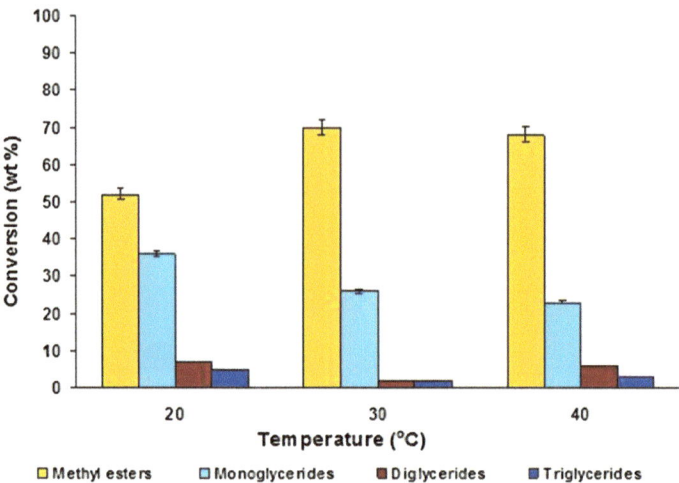

Fig. 4.16 Effect of temperature on immobilized lipase catalyzed transesterification of palm oil (Process conditions: 5.25 g of immobilized lipase, 10 g of oil, 2.5 g of methanol, 1 g water a stirring rate of $14.3 \times g$ RCF and a 24 h reaction) (Jegannathan et al. 2010)

4.5.4 Effect of Temperature

The reaction rate increases with temperature to a maximum level, then declines with further increase of temperature in enzymatic reactions. Figure 4.16 shows the transesterification activity of immobilized lipase with variations in temperature. The optimum temperature was found to be 30 °C. Above this temperature there was no significant increase in methyl ester formation. The production of biodiesel at milder temperature is an advantage of enzymatic reactions which can save lot of energy in the production unit. In literature, biodiesel production using immobilized lipase, at the temperature range 30–50 °C have been reported (Wang et al. 2006; Yang et al. 2006). Kumari et al. (2007) has reported an optimum temperature at 40 °C. In support to this work Watanabe et al. (2001) and Samukawa et al. (2000) has reported the optimum temperature at 30 °C. The reason for this difference in temperatures could be due to the type of matrix, the source of enzyme used and other reaction conditions. Thus, biodiesel production at near room temperature is a major advantage of using enzymatic catalyst. This could bring considerable energy savings in the biodiesel process industry and also favours the environment.

4.5.5 Effect of Reaction Time

The reaction time study result of transesterification reaction of palm oil with methanol is shown in (Fig. 4.17). The highest methyl esters formation was observed at 72 h reaction time and the conversion remained static with further increase in

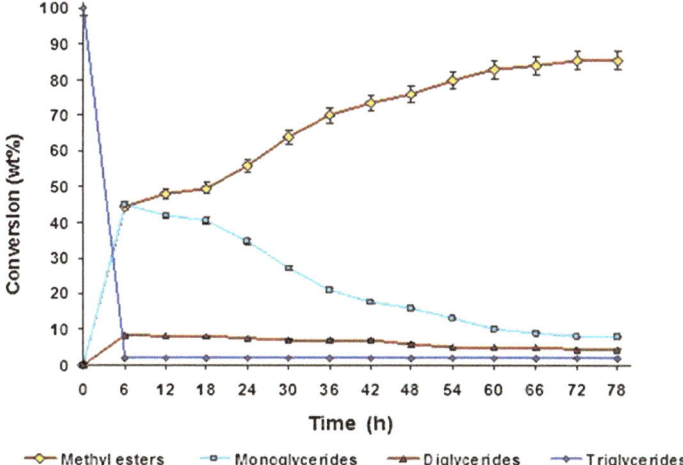

Fig. 4.17 Effect of time course on immobilized lipase catalyzed transesterification of palm oil (Process condition: 5.25 g of immobilized lipase, 10 g of oil, 2.5 g of methanol, 1 g water and a stirring rate of $14.3 \times g$ RCF at 30 °C) (Jegannathan et al. 2010)

reaction time. At the end of 6 h the formation of 44.5 % methyl esters and 45 % monoglycerides were observed. At the end of 72 h methyl ester and monoglycerides formation was found to be 85.5 % and 10 % respectively. This reveals that immobilized PS lipase converts the first two steps of the transesterification reaction of triglycerides to monoglycerides faster and the third step, the monoglycerides to methyl esters at a slower rate.

In the literature, Yagiz et al. (2007) has reported a reaction time of 105 h for conversion above 95 % and Orcaire et al. (2006) reported 360 h for 39 % conversion using the same lipase immobilized in a different carrier. The reason for lower methyl ester conversion (85.5 %) could be due to the diffusion limitations caused by the immobilization matrix. This is because, when enzymes encapsulated in porous matrix, substrate diffuses through the tortuous pathway inside the pores of the external membrane and react with the enzyme (Schuler and Kargi 1992).

4.5.6   Effect of Mixing Intensity

The effect of mixing intensity on transesterification results shown in Fig. 4.18 revealed that increase in methyl ester conversion was observed as the mixing intensity increased. At $23.7 \times g$ (RCF) (450 rpm) the methyl ester conversion reached near to 100 %. Mixing intensity plays a major role in the immobilized enzyme systems with respect to diffusion and reaction rate. The diffusion limitations in immobilized enzyme reactions can be eliminated either by decreasing the immobilized

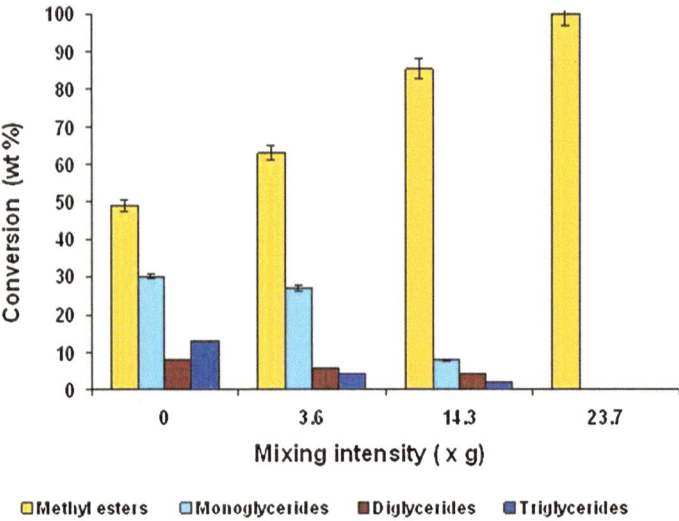

Fig. 4.18 Effect of mixing intensity on immobilized lipase catalyzed transesterification of palm oil (Process conditions: 5.25 g of immobilized lipase, 10 g of oil, 2.5 g of methanol, 1 g water and a 72 h reaction at 30 °C) (Jegannathan et al. 2010)

enzyme particle size or by creating a higher degree of turbulence around the particle (Schuler and Kargi 1992). However, higher mixing intensity may also lead to immobilized enzyme rupture.

In literature, the effect of mixing intensity in the optimization of biodiesel production using immobilized lipase has been reported by Halim and Kamaruddin (2008). With an increase in speed from 140 rpm to 200 rpm, the FAME yield was found to increase. The highest FAME yield of 88 % was obtained at 200 rpm (Halim and Kamaruddin 2008). Various authors have reported the methyl ester conversion in a fixed mixing intensity. Wang et al. (2006) has reported 97 % conversion at 150 rpm/min and Sung et al. (2007) has reported 80 % conversion at 250 rpm/min where as Noureddini et al. (2005) has reported 56.5 % conversion at 700 rpm/min. Similarly, Salis et al. (2005) has reported > 99 % and 100 % conversion at 150 and 80 rpm/min respectively. These contrary reports on mixing intensity leads to the conclusion that, the mixing intensity depends on the individual reaction system.

4.5.7 Reusability of Immobilized Enzyme

The reusability study of immobilized enzyme in the transesterification of palm oil with methanol is shown in Fig. 4.19. The transesterification activity decreased gradually for each recycle and relative methyl ester conversion of 45 % could be observed after 10 reuses. The decrease in transesterification activity of immobilized lipase upon reuse has been reported by most of the authors in literature. The decrease in methyl esters conversion upon reuse might be due to the leakage of enzyme from

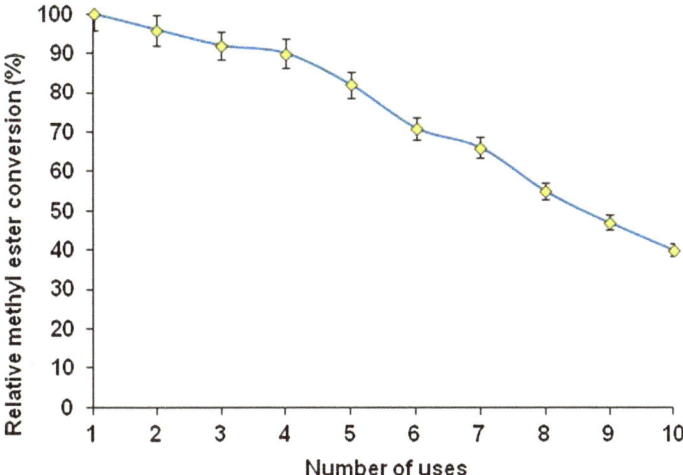

Fig. 4.19 Reusability of immobilized lipase (Process conditions: 5.25 g of immobilized lipase, 10 g of oil, 2.5 g of methanol, 1 g water, 23.7×g RCF and a 72 h reaction at 30 °C) (Jegannathan et al. 2010)

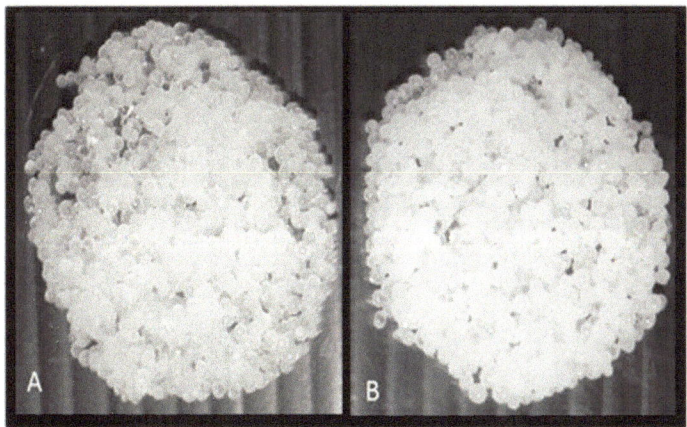

Fig. 4.20 κ-carrageenen encapsulated lipase (**a**) before and (**b**) after 10 uses in transesterification of palm oil with methanol at 23.7×g RCF and 30 °C (Jegannathan et al. 2009)

the matrix (Yadav and Jadhav 2005) or due to the blockage of pores in the matrix by the glycerol formed during transesterification (Watanabe et al. 2000; Jegannathan et al. 2008). Thus, leakage of enzyme from the immobilized catalyst is a major problem in bioprocess system. Avoiding leakage of enzyme upon reuse is a challenging task in immobilized enzyme system and it could be an important area to work in the future.

The encapsulated lipase in κ-carrageenan was reused in transesterification reaction for 10 cycles (720 h) at 23.7×g RCF in a baffled flask; the capsules did not show any deformation in their physical structure (Fig. 4.20). The possible reason for this kind of behaviour from encapsulated lipase could be the action of methanol and glycerol on κ-carrageeenan matrix. This claim is confirmed by the previous reports (Tosa et al. 1979; Winston et al. 1994) showing the increase κ-carragenen matrix gel strength with methanol and glycerol. Thus, κ-carrageenan would be a promising matrix for lipase immobilization in biodiesel production using methanol as solvent, but still decrease in activity.

4.6   Production of Biodiesel Using Immobilized Lipase in Recirculated Packed Bed Immobilized Bioreactor

The process parameters in a packed bed bioreactor are similar to the immobilized batch bioreactor. In the literature (Rayon et al. 2007; Watanabe et al. 2000; Samukawa et al. 2000; Du et al. 2005; Lu et al. 2007) have reported that the flow rate and the reaction time were the significant parameters for biodiesel in packed bed reactor.

4.6.1   Effect of Flow Rate

The effect of flow rate (down flow) on biodiesel production is shown in Fig. 4.21. It can be observed that the methyl ester production was a direct function of flow rate with maximum methyl ester conversion at a flow rate of 1.5 ml/min.

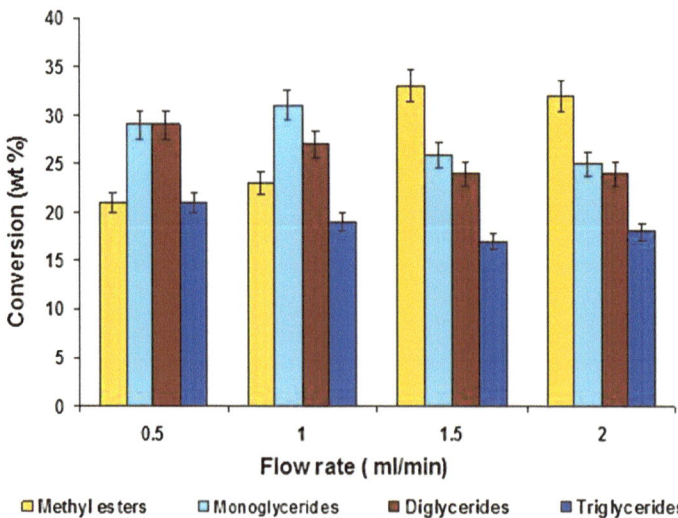

Fig. 4.21 Effect of flow rate on immobilized lipase catalyzed transesterification of palm oil (Process conditions: Palm oil to alcohol mole ratio of 1:7, palm oil 40 g, 21 g immobilized lipase and 4 g water at 30 °C)

Accordingly, at 1.5 ml/min, methyl ester conversion of 33 % was observed for 24 h reaction time. When the flow rate was increased further, pressure drop in the reactor increased drastically leading to back flow. In literature, Watanabe et al. (2000) has reported 91.6 % methyl ester conversion at a flow rate of 4.1 ml/min using immobilized lipase by adsorption method. Whereas, Rayon et al. (2007) has reported 95 % conversion at 0.16 ml/min, Halim et al. (2009) has reported 79 % yield at 0.57 ml/min. Thus, the flow rate depends on the immobilized enzyme used and the reaction system configuration.

4.6.2   Effect of Reaction Time

Figure 4.22 shows the conversion of triglycerides to methyl esters catalyzed by immobilized PS lipase with respect to reaction time. At the end of 264 h methyl esters conversion of 86 % could be observed. This was very low compared to the conversion achieved by Watanabe et al. (2000), Rayon et al. (2007) and Halim and Kamaruddin (2008). The reason for lower methyl ester conversion could be due to the lack of intensive agitation in packed bed immobilized reactor leading to low diffusion of substrate and products in the encapsulated lipase. Hence it can be concluded that the efficiency of the encapsulated lipase is very low in packed bed immobilized bioreactor compared to stirred tank immobilized bioreactor.

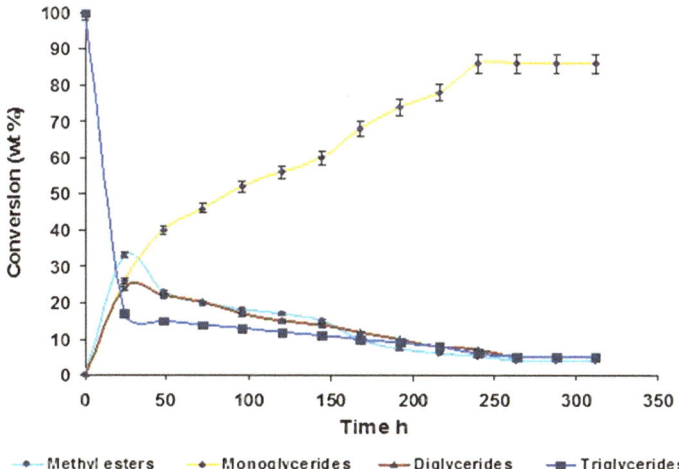

Fig. 4.22 Effect of reaction time on immobilized lipase catalyzed transesterification of palm oil (Process conditions: Palm oil -to-alcohol mole ratio of 1:7, palm oil 40 g, 21 g immobilized lipase, 4 g water and 1.5 ml/min flow rate at 30 °C)

Process parameters	Stirred tank bioreactor	Packed bed bioreactor
Oil:methanol ratio	1:7	1:7
Water content	1 % of oil w/w	1 % of oil w/w
Enzyme loading	4.2 % of oil w/w	4.2 % of oil w/w
Temperature	30 °C	30 °C
Mixing intensity	23.7×g	–
Flow rate	–	1.5 ml/min
Reaction time	72 h	264 h
Conversion	100 %	86 %

Table 4.6 Comparison of biodiesel production in immobilized bioreactors

4.6.3   Comparison of Biodiesel Production in Stirred Tank Immobilized Bioreactor With Recirculated Packed Bed Immobilized Bioreactor

The optimization studies revealed that the biodiesel production using encapsulated lipase was relatively better in stirred tank immobilized bioreactor compared to recirculated packed bed immobilized bioreactor under similar process conditions. Table 4.6. shows the optimized conditions, the methyl ester conversion and the reaction time for packed bed bioreactor was poor compared to the stirred tank bioreactor. The possible reason for this could be the lack of mixing in the packed bed reactor. In literature, biodiesel conversion in the range of 87.4–98.7 % and reaction time in the range 3.5–48 h has been reported for packed bed immobilized bioreactor (Rayon et al. 2007; Watanabe et al. 2000; Samukawa et al. 2000; Du et al. 2005; Lu et al. 2007). Where as in stirred tank immobilized bioreactor, biodiesel conversion in the range of 64–100 % and reaction time in the range 2.5–300 h has been reported (Iso et al. 2001; Shah et al. 2004).

4.7   Kinetics and Modelling of Biodiesel Production Using Encapsulated Lipase

The optimization of biodiesel production using encapsulated lipase results revealed that batch reactor shows higher methyl ester conversion compared to the packed bed reactor for the same set of reaction conditions. Hence, the reaction kinetics was studied for biodiesel production in stirred tank batch reactor using encapsulated lipase.

In literature, kinetics of biodiesel production using immobilized lipase has been reported by several researchers. They have considered the multi substrate reactions (Xu et al. 2005; Dossat et al. 2002; Al-Zuhair 2005; Halim and Kamaruddin 2008). Since the results obtained by the different investigators was similar to the results of the single substrate reactions as observed by our work. Therefore, in this study the single substrate reaction is considered in an attempt to represent the experimental kinetic data in a batch reactor. A simplified reaction mechanism was proposed by considering the equation (4.1).

$$T + E \underset{K_1}{\overset{K_2}{\Longleftrightarrow}} TE \overset{K_3}{\longrightarrow} ME + E \tag{4.1}$$

Where, T stands for triglycerides (substrate), E for enzyme and TE for substrate enzyme complex, ME for methyl esters respectively.

The following assumptions have been made:

  (i) reversible reaction
 (ii) no loss of enzyme activity during reaction
(iii) no mass-transfer limitations
 (iv) no intermediate reaction products, mono- and diglycerides
  (v) The above reaction obeys Michaelis Menten equation.

The velocity of an enzyme-catalyzed reaction can be determined from the disappearance of substrate (−d[S]/dt) as a function of time (Alejandro 2003). For a constant volume batch reactor, the Michaelis Menten equation gives a form of an equation that can be linearized as

$$\left(+r_p\right) = \left(-r_s\right) = \frac{-dC_s}{dt} = \frac{V_{max} C_S}{K_m + C_S} \tag{4.2}$$

Rearranging equation (4.2) gives

$$\left(K_m + C_S\right) \frac{dC_S}{C_S} = -V_{max} dt \tag{4.3}$$

$$-K_m \frac{dC_S}{C_S} - dC_S = dC_S = V_{max} dt \tag{4.4}$$

Integrating equation (4.3) with the boundary conditions $C_S = C_{SO}$ at $t = 0$ gives

$$-K_m \ln\left(\frac{C_S}{C_{SO}}\right) - \left(C_S - C_{SO}\right) = V_{max} dt \tag{4.5}$$

Equation 4.4 can further be rearranged to give (Kayode Coker 2001)

$$\frac{1}{t} \ln\left(\frac{C_{SO}}{C_S}\right) = \frac{V_{max}}{K_m} - \frac{1}{K_m}\left(\frac{C_S - C_{SO}}{t}\right) \tag{4.6}$$

Where,

$+r_p$ = rate of product formation (Methyl esters)
$-r_s$ = rate of disappearance of substrate (Triglycerides)
C_S = concentration of the substrate at time t
C_{SO} = concentration of the substrate at time $t = 0$

Table 4.7 Experimental studies of biodiesel production using encapsulated lipase in stirred tank batch reactor (Time vs Concentration)

Time (min)	Substrate conc. (%)	C_{S0} (Mol/m³)	C_S (Mol/m³)	$\ln(C_{S0}/C_S)$	$C_{S0}-C_S/t$	$1/t$ $\ln(C_{S0}/C_S)$
0	100	940	940	–	–	–
360	56	940	526.4	0.579818	1.14888	0.00161
720	43	940	404.2	0.84397	0.74416	0.00117
1,080	33	940	310.2	1.108663	0.58314	0.00102
1,440	21	940	197.4	1.560648	0.51569	0.00108
1,800	18	940	169.2	1.714798	0.42822	0.00095
2,160	16	940	150.4	1.832581	0.36555	0.00084
2,520	12	940	112.8	2.120264	0.32825	0.00084
2,880	6	940	56.4	2.813411	0.30680	0.00097
3,240	5	940	47	2.995732	0.27561	0.00092
3,600	3	940	28.2	3.506558	0.25327	0.00097
3,960	2	940	18.8	3.912023	0.23262	0.00098
4,320	1	940	9.4	4.60517	0.21541	0.00106

Equation (4.4) shows $1/t \ln (C_{S0}/C_S)$ as a linear function of $(C_{S0} - C_S)/t$. The parameters K_m and V_{max} can be estimated from Equation (4.4) using measured values of C_S as a function of t for a given C_{S0}. Table 4.7 shows the corresponding plot in terms of substrate concentration. When the kinetic constants, the initial concentration of substrate, and the desired conversions are known, the required batch time t can be calculated.

$$t = \frac{K_m}{V_{max}} \ln\left(\frac{C_{S0}}{C_S}\right) + \left(\frac{C_{S0} - C_S}{V_{max}}\right) \tag{4.7}$$

From the Fig. (4.23)

$$V_{max} = 0.84\left(\text{mol}/\text{m}^3.\text{min}\right)$$

$$K_m = 600\left(\text{mol}/\text{m}^3\right)$$

$$t = 712.28\ln\left(\frac{C_{S0}}{C_S}\right) + \left(\frac{C_{S0} - C_S}{8.2 \times 10^{-7}}\right) \tag{4.8}$$

From the experimental studies the kinetic parameters K_m and V_{max} were determined to be $K_m = 600$ (mol/m³) $V_{max} = 0.84$ (mol/m³.min). Whereas the Kcat (Turn over number) value with an initial enzyme concentration of 0.48 (mol/m³) was found to be 1.75. The value of K_{cat} for palm oil transesterification reaction was found to be very low compared to the p-NPP hydrolysis reaction. Thus, the transesterification

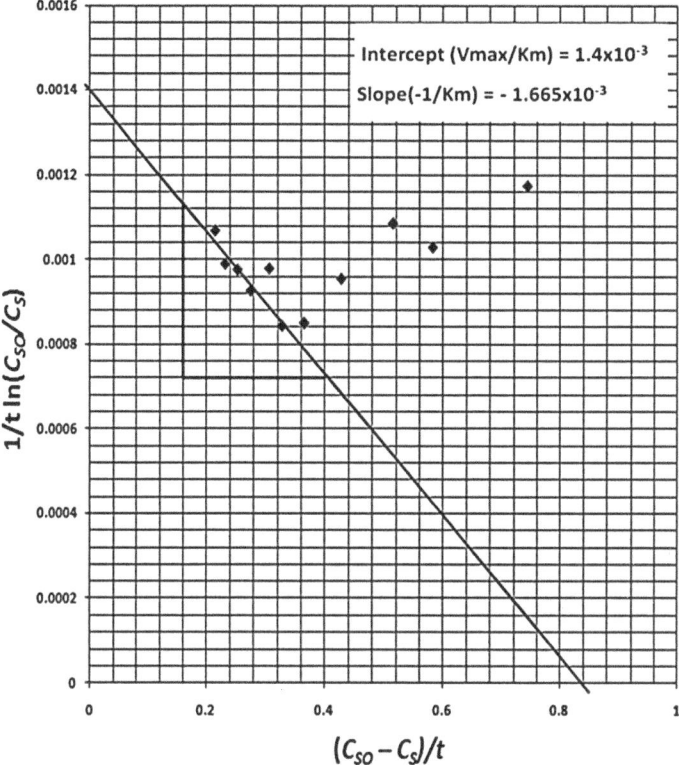

Fig. 4.23 Estimation of K_m and V_{max}

reaction tends to be very slow compared to hydrolysis. Both first order and second order was observed in the transesterification reaction (Fig. 4.24). The reaction followed first order trend until 48 h and later pseudo second order trend was observed. The reason for this kind of behaviour was, in the initial reaction time the concentration of the substrate and the enzyme was too high leading to first order trend in the later stage the decrease in the substrate leads to low binding of enzyme to the substrate following pseudo second order.

An empirical model equation for biodiesel production using the kinetic parameters in stirred tank bioreactor was derived (Equation 4.8). The predicted model showed fair agreement with the experimental data for the first order trend in the initial reaction time and good agreement with the pseudo second order trend in the final reaction time (Fig. 4.24). When the initial concentration of substrate and the desired conversions are known, the required batch time t can thus easily be calculated using the model equation. Figure 4.25 shows the validation of the model with $R^2 = 0.9393$ indicating a deviation of 6.07 %.

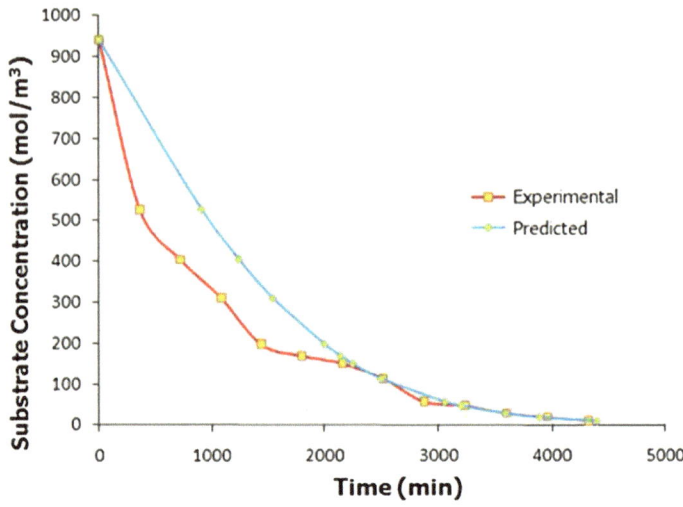

Fig. 4.24 Comparison of required batch time (Predicted and Experimental)

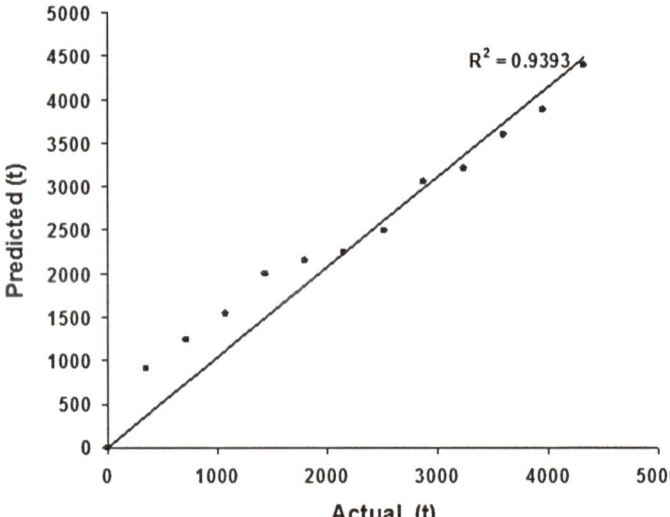

Fig. 4.25 Validation of the model

4.7.1 Diffusion Effect of κ-Carrageenan Encapsulated Lipase in Biodiesel Production

In the kinetic study it has been assumed that there is no mass transfer limitation in the reaction system. The significance of mass transfer limitations in a reaction system using immobilized lipase can be shown using the effectiveness factor. The effectiveness factor (η) is defined as the ratio of the reaction with diffusion limitation to the reaction rate with no diffusion limitation. The value of the effectiveness factor is a measure of the extent of diffusion limitation.

For $\eta < 1$ the conversion is mass transfer controlled, whereas for $\eta \approx 1$, the conversion is limited by reaction rate and diffusion limitations are negligible. The factor is a function of Φ (Thiele modulus) and β (Schuler and Kargi 1992).

Where,

$$\eta = \frac{3}{\Phi}\left(\frac{1}{\tanh \Phi} - \frac{1}{\Phi}\right) (\text{Schuler and Kargi} 1992) \tag{4.9}$$

$$\Phi = r\frac{\sqrt{V''\frac{m}{Km}}}{De} (\text{Schuler and Kargi} 1992) \tag{4.10}$$

$$De = \frac{KT}{6\pi r}\frac{1}{\mu} (\text{Griffiths} 1995) \tag{4.11}$$

$$\beta = \frac{km}{S0} (\text{Schuler and Kargi} 1992) \tag{4.12}$$

Substituting the parameter values (Table 4.8) into the equations 4.8,4.9,4.10 and 4.11 the η, Φ, β, De were found to be

De	1.96×10^{-17} m²/s
Φ -	2.39
β -	0.625
η -	0.75

From the calculated value Φ and the Fig. 4.26, the effective factor for this system using encapsulated lipase was found to be 0.75 and tends towards 1. Thus, the diffusion limitation in this study is insignificant and can be neglected. The reason for the lack of diffusion limitation can be explained by the smaller size of the encapsulated lipase and the high mixing intensity.

Table 4.8 Values of the parameters for effectiveness factor (η) determination

Parameter	Values	Remarks
V_m''	1.68×10^{-6} mol/m³ (catalyst). sec	Apparent maximum reaction rate calculated from the maximum reaction rate.
K_m	600 mol/ m³	Michaelis Menten constant
K	1.38×10^{-23} kg m²/s²	Boltzmann constant
T	303 K	Reaction temperature
$r = (r_1 - r_2)$	2×10^{-4} m	r_1, r_2 are the outer and inner core radius of the capsule
μ	0.056 kg/m.s	Viscosity of substrate
So	940 mol/ mol/m³	Initial substrate concentration

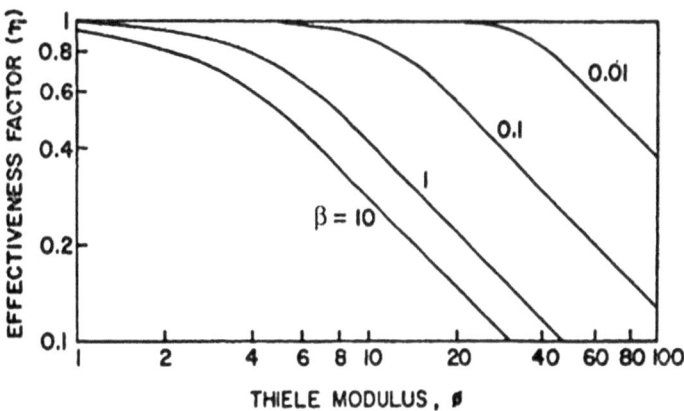

Fig. 4.26 Theoretical relation between the effectiveness factor η, the modules Φ and β (Schuler and Kargi 1992)

4.8 Catalytic and Non-Catalytic Functions of κ-Carrageenan Encapsulated Lipase

Immobilized enzyme has to meet three essential functions, namely the catalytic function that are designed to convert the substrate to required product, the non-catalytic function designed to aid separation and the environment friendly factor to achieve sustainability.

4.8.1 Catalytic Function

Catalytic function is an important factor for an immobilized enzyme to achieve its target in production process. Transesterification activity up to 100 % was achieved by employing the immobilized lipase at an optimized condition of 5.25 g of immobilized lipase, 10 g of oil, 2.5 g of methanol, 1 g water, and 72 h reaction time at 30 °C. This result confirms that the process parameters involved in lipase immobilization did not alter the activity of the enzyme. Similarly, the κ-carrageenan matrix used for immobilizing lipase did not show any adverse effect on the catalytic activity of lipase enzyme. In literature, the catalytic function of immobilized lipase produced via various methods and various matrices have been reported in several reviews and the catalytic activity in transesterification reaction ranges from 3 to 100 % (Akoh et al. 2007; Jegannathan et al. 2008) The reason for this drastic difference could be due the different process parameters and immobilized enzymes preparation from various sources and matrices.

Burkholderia cepacia immobilized lipase produced using Diatomaceous earth (Salis et al. 2005) and Celite (Shah and Gupta 2006) via adsorption method, Glutaraldehyde (Kumari et al. 2007) via cross-linkage, Phyllosilicate sol-gel (Noureddini et al. 2005) and Hydrophobic sol-gel (Hsu et al. 2001) via entrapment has shown catalytic activity in the range of 91–100 % conversion in biodiesel production. But *Burkholderia cepacia* lipase encapsulated in silica aero gel (Orcaire et al. 2006) has shown only 64 % conversion.

4.8.2 Isolation of Catalyst from the Application Environment

In biodiesel production, where a high viscosity raw material is involved, agglomeration of immobilized enzyme particles should be avoided for easy reuse of immobilized enzyme and separation of product. This can be achieved by immobilizing enzyme with precise size and shape. In this study, encapsulated lipase with definite particle size and shape was produced by co-extrusion technique. The encapsulated lipase enzyme was found to be spherical in shape with the size range of 1.3 to 1.8 mm in diameter. The immobilized enzyme did not show any agglomeration and the isolation of the catalyst from reaction mixture was easily achieved by simple filtration process using a sieve with mesh no 20. Unfortunately, in literature the immobilized enzyme size and the agglomeration of catalyst are not reported in biodiesel production. But In general, the size of immobilized enzyme prepared via adsorption, cross linkage and covalent bonding method are very small ranging from 50 to 300 μm which may agglomerate and lead to difficulty in reuse of the immobilized lipase. However, by entrapment and by encapsulation methods, higher size range of immobilized enzymes (in mm) can be prepared favouring easy reusability and avoiding agglomeration.

4.8.3 Stability

Chemical and mechanical stability of the immobilized catalyst also plays a major role in production process. It is important to ensure that the immobilized catalyst used is compatible with all raw material and products formed; do not contaminate the products and the by-products. Biodiesel production from palm oil transesterification involves palm oil, methanol, and water as raw materials, methyl esters, and glycerol as product and by-product. Lipase encapsulated in κ-carrageenan by coextrusion technique did not show any adverse effect on any of the materials used. This reveals that the immobilized enzyme use in this study is stable and compatible with the raw materials, product and by-product. In addition, the raw material methanol (Tosa et al. 1979) and the by-product glycerol (Winston et al. 1994) in this process favour to strengthen the κ-carrageenan gel matrix. The increase in mechanical strength of the capsules was also found by observation while handling the capsules.

The possible reason could be that, the contact of κ-carrageenan with methanol and glycerol increase the gel strength. This additional effect contributed by methanol and glycerol is an advantage of using κ-carrageenan as a matrix in biodiesel production process.

4.8.4   Eco-Friendly Factors

In recent years the concept of eco-friendly factor is gaining importance in all the fields to ensure sustainability. Use of renewable and biodegradable materials with milder process is important to attain the eco-friendly factor. κ-carrageenan, is an anionic, hydrophilic, most abundant and naturally occurring polysaccharide found in numerous species of seaweed. Chemically, it is a linear, sulphated polysaccharide, composed of repeating units of β-D-galactose sulfate and 3, 6-anhydro β-d-galactose. κ-carrageenan is mainly used as gelling, thickening and stabilizing agent due to its biocompatibility, biodegradability, and mechanical strength. In addition, the milder conditions of immobilization and the biodiesel production process also favour eco-friendly factors. The matrices used for lipase immobilization in biodiesel production like Glutaraldehyde, Hydrophobic sol-gel, Phyllosilicate sol-gel, Silica aerogel, Silica-PVA, Celite and Diatomaceous earth are not biodegradable and hence would cause disposal problems when used in large scale production of biodiesel. Thus the biodegradable property of κ-carrageenan encapsulated lipase makes this biocatalyst a superior immobilized enzyme for biodiesel production. Further, unlike other matrices, the κ-carrageenan encapsulated lipase after using for several times, in biodiesel production can also be reutilized as biomass in anaerobic fermentation for energy production. This may generate additional revenue for the biodiesel industry and also avoids catalyst disposal problems.

4.9   Life Cycle Assessment (LCA) of Biodiesel Production

Figures 4.27, 4.28, and 4.29 shows the life cycle impacts (the effect of raw materials, product and the process used on environment). 1,000 kg palm biodiesel capacity of alkali-catalyzed process showed a lower environmental impact by low values of carcinogens, respiratory organics, respiratory inorganic, land use and acidification. When the size of the production capacity increased the number of categories showing lower impact increased further (Fig. 4.28). In 10,000 kg production capacity the alkali catalyst process showed higher impact for 6 categories out of 11 compared to the other two processes (shown as percentage release of the impact categories) in Fig. 4.29, particularly the impact on the radiation and ozone layer were higher; this could be due to the usage of hazardous materials such as sodium hydroxide and hydrochloric acid by the alkali catalyst process. Similar trend was followed for the impact on human health, ecosystem and resources. Thes results were similar to that of Harding et al. (2008).

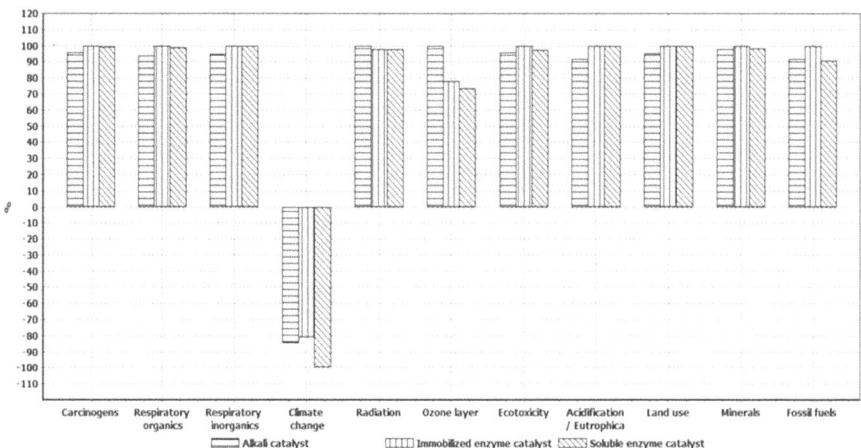

Fig. 4.27 Comparison of the environmental impacts on each of the 11 environmental categories due to the production of 1,000 kg palm biodiesel (Jegannathan et al. 2011b)

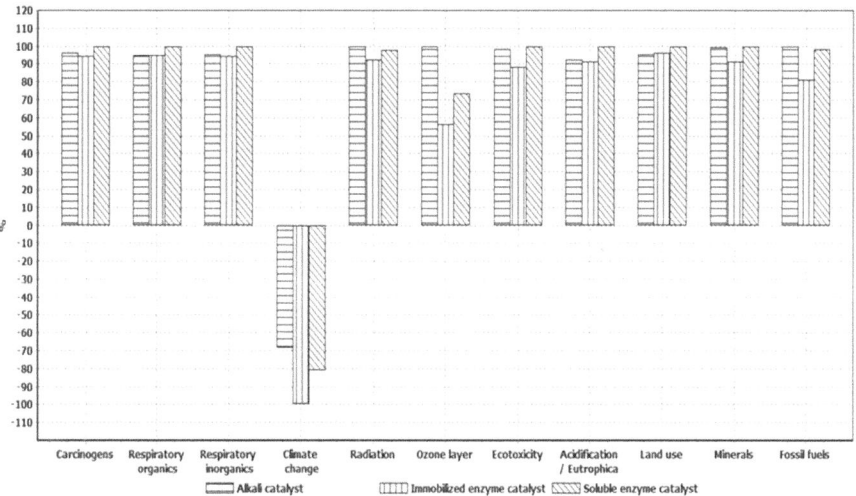

Fig. 4.28 Comparison of the environmental impacts biodiesel on each of the 11 environmental categories due to the production of 5,000 kg palm biodiesel (Jegannathan et al. 2011b)

In biodiesel production using soluble enzyme catalyst process, as the production capacity increased from 1,000 kg (Fig. 4.30) to 10,000 kg (Fig. 4.31) the impact level was equal to that of alkali catalyst. This is because in the soluble enzyme catalyst process two production units are involved namely the biodiesel production and the lipase production unit which leads to high consumption of energy and raw materials. However, the impact on radiation, ozone layer and climate change remained less compared to the alkali catalyst. This is because the soluble enzyme process does not use hazardous materials such as sodium hydroxide and hydrochloric acid.

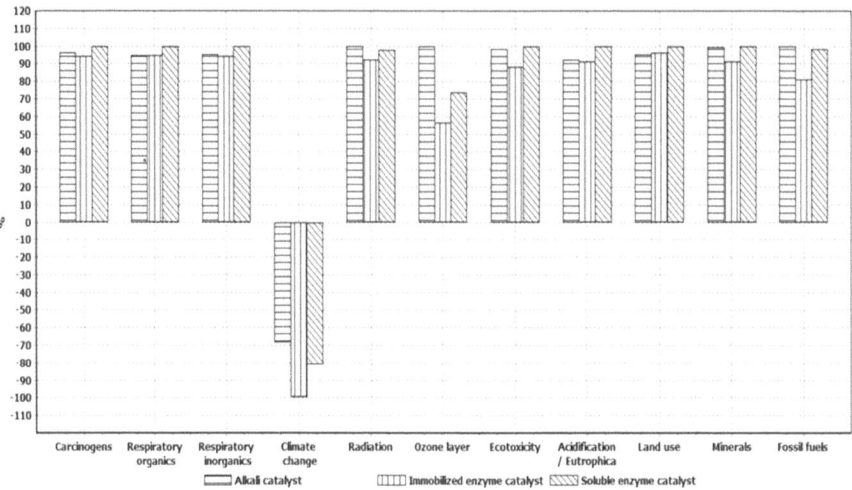

Fig. 4.29 Comparison of the environmental impacts on each of the 11 environmental categories due to the production of 10,000 kg palm biodiesel (Jegannathan et al. 2011b)

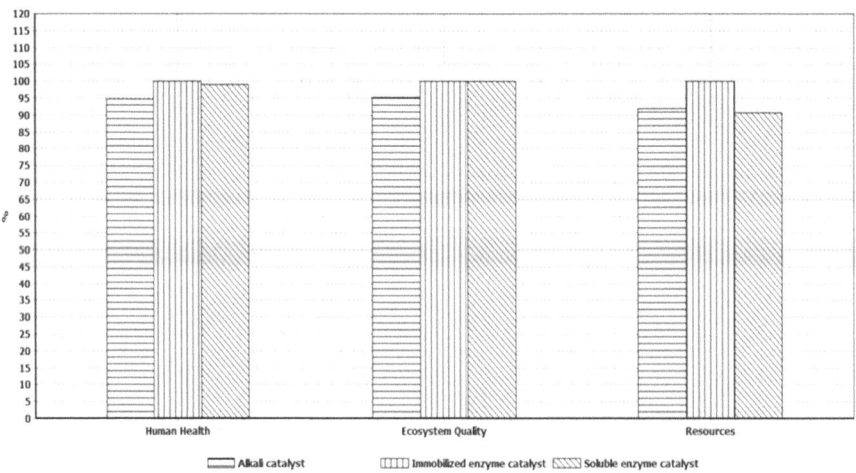

Fig. 4.30 Comparison of the environmental impacts on human health, ecosystem and resources due to the production of 1,000 kg palm biodiesel (Jegannathan et al. 2011b)

Whereas, the impact on human health, ecosystem and resources were also showed higher as the production capacity increased from 1,000 kg to 10,000 kg. The reason for this increase in the impact could be that, the soluble enzyme catalyst cannot be reused hence the catalyst has to be produced for each batch of 1,000 kg biodiesel production involving higher raw materials and energy consumption (Fig. 4.32).

Out of 11, 8 categories were showing higher impact for 1,000 kg biodiesel production unit using immobilized catalyst. The reason for the higher impact could be that,

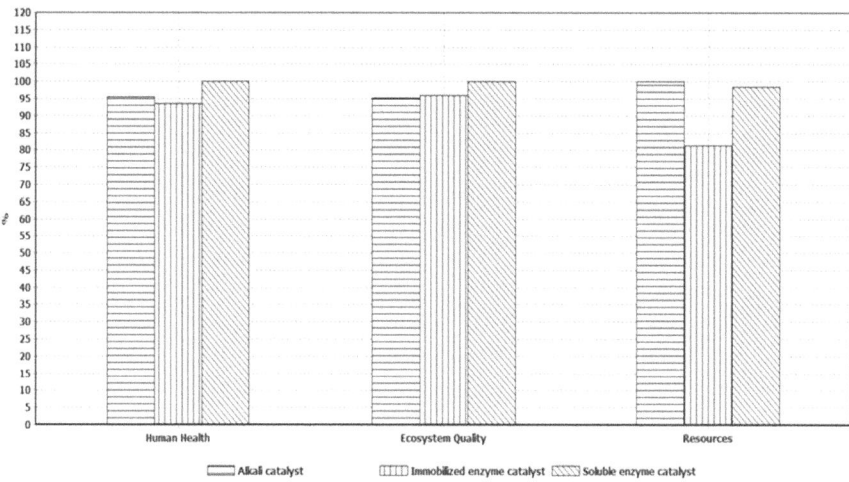

Fig. 4.31 Comparison of the environmental impacts on human health, ecosystem and resources due to the production of 5,000 kg palm biodiesel (Jegannathan et al. 2011b)

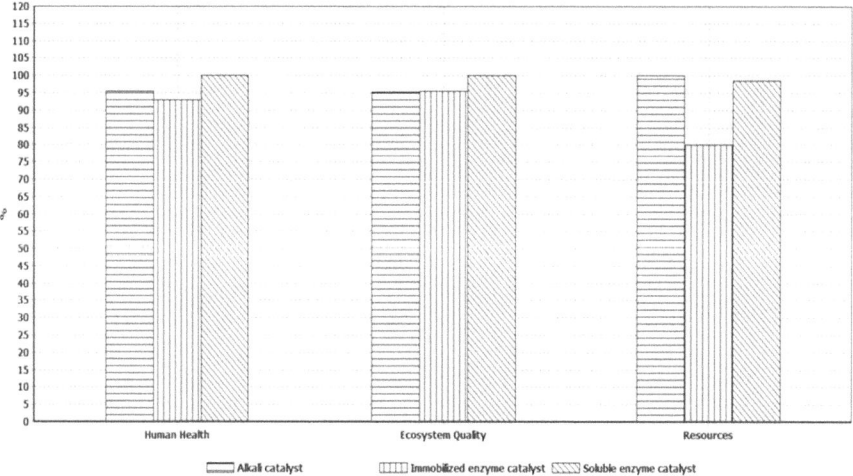

Fig. 4.32 Comparison of the environmental impacts on human health, ecosystem and resources due to the production of 10,000 kg palm biodiesel (Jegannathan et al. 2011b)

the biodiesel production using immobilized enzyme catalyst involves 3 production units namely; κ-carrageenan, lipase and biodiesel. Hence the raw materials and the energy used were more compared to the other two processes, Similar to the soluble enzyme catalyst process the impact on radiations and ozone layer were less compared to the alkali catalyst process. These higher impacts were decreased on further increase in the production capacity (Figs. 4.29, 4.30) and since the immobilized

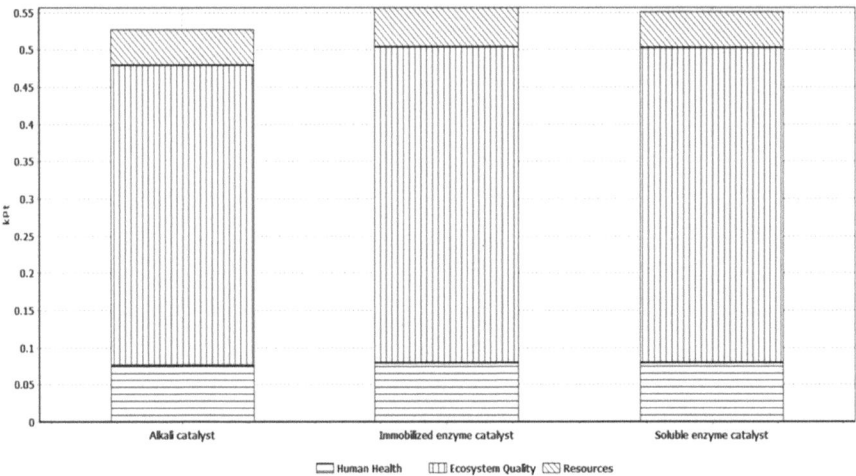

Fig. 4.33 Comparison of the environmental impacts on each environmental category based on a single cumulative score due to the production of 1,000 kg palm biodiesel (Jegannathan et al. 2011b)

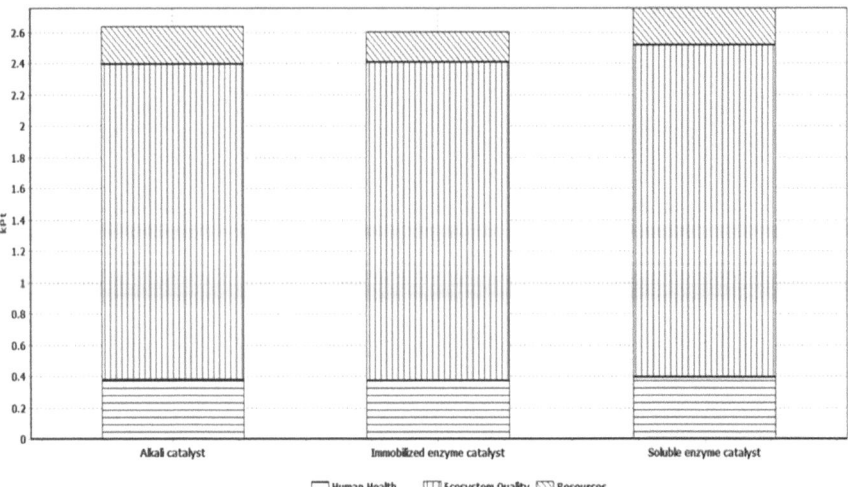

Fig. 4.34 Comparison of the environmental impacts on each environmental category based on a single cumulative score due to the production of 5,000 kg palm biodiesel (Jegannathan et al. 2011b)

enzyme could be reused, the raw materials, energy for the lipase production unit and κ-carrageenan unit could be saved resulting in lower impact on environment. For 10,000 kg biodiesel production unit using immobilized lipase, the environmental impacts were lower for all the 11 categories (Fig. 4.29). The impact on human health, ecosystem and resources were also lessened when the biodiesel production capacity increased from 1,000 to 10,000 kg (Figs. 4.33, 4.34, and 4.35). Thus, the LCA results

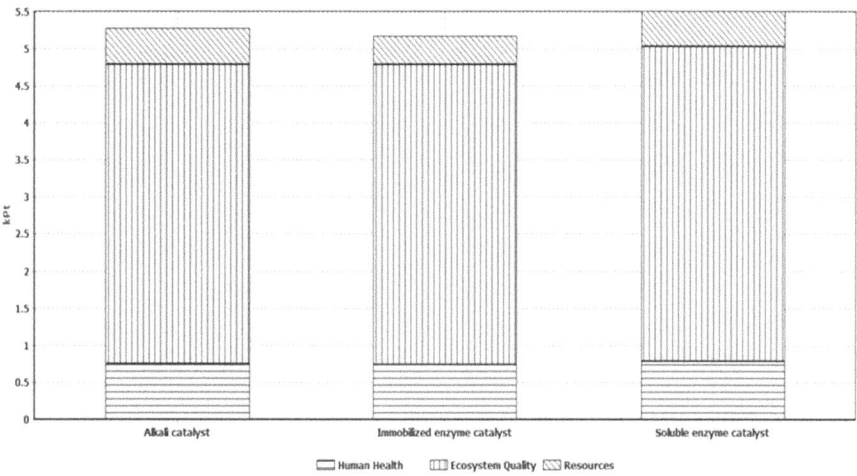

Fig. 4.35 Comparison of the environmental impacts on each environmental category based on a single cumulative score due to the production of 10,000 kg palm biodiesel (Jegannathan et al. 2011b)

has shown the significant of using immobilized enzyme catalyst compared to that of alkali and soluble enzyme catalyst in biodiesel production.

The key factor in the immobilized lipase lies in the usage of natural products and the capacity of the immobilized enzyme to be reused several times. As on now only one study has been reported on the Life cycle assessment on biodiesel production using immobilized lipase (Harding et al. 2008). Unfortunately, the raw materials and the energy requirement for enzyme production and immobilization was not considered in the inventory analysis. However, in this work those points were taken into consideration. Thus, the life cycle assessment results of this report may be a fore front for the future lifecycle assessment studies.

4.10 Economic Assessment of Biodiesel Production

Figures 4.36 and 4.37 shows the plant cost (per 1,000 tonnes), manufacturing cost (per tonne) for biodiesel production process using different catalysts. From the figures it can observed that, the plant cost for biodiesel production using immobilized enzyme was 57.18 % higher than the alkali catalyst process and 0.40 % higher than soluble enzyme catalyst process. The high cost for both the soluble and immobilized catalyst process was due to the process time variation with respect to the alkali catalyst. To achieve the process time equal to the alkali chemical catalyst, the enzymatic catalyst process was calculated to operate 5 units. Hence the plant cost for the enzymatic process has increased drastically compared to the alkali chemical catalyst biodiesel production process. Likewise, a marginal increase of plant cost for immobilized catalyst process over soluble enzyme process was due to the addition of encapsulation unit, which has caused a 0.4 % increase.

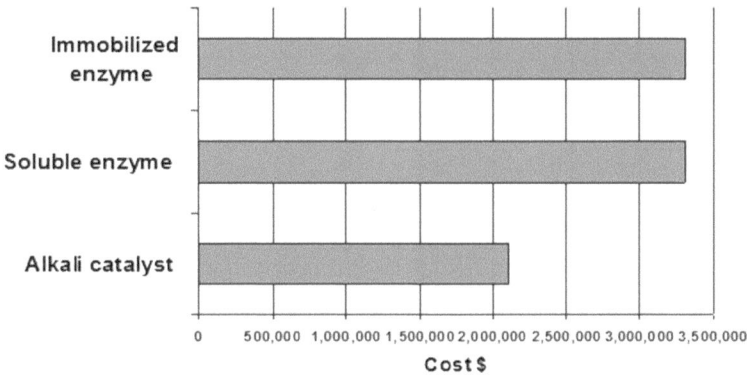

Fig. 4.36 Plant investment costs for 1,000 tonnes capacity biodiesel production (Jegannathan et al. 2011a)

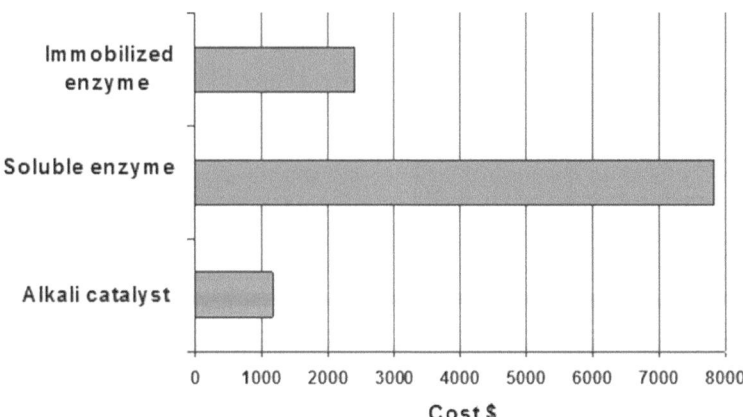

Fig. 4.37 Manufacturing costs for 1 tonne capacity biodiesel production (Jegannathan et al. 2011b)

The manufacturing cost (per tonne) of immobilized enzyme catalyst process was 206.96 % higher than alkali catalyst process and 323.9 % lesser than the soluble enzyme catalyst process. The higher manufacturing cost of enzyme catalyst process over alkali catalyst process was due to the cost of lipase enzyme for soluble enzyme catalyst and the cost of lipase enzyme and κ-carrageenan for immobilized enzyme catalyst process. Whereas, the reason was lesser manufacturing cost of immobilized enzyme catalyst over soluble enzyme catalyst was the ability to reuse immobilized enzyme catalyst. However it is expected that the enzyme cost would reduce in the years to come due to drastic development in the white biotechnology in various country around the world.

4.11   Conclusion

The conventional production of biodiesel by chemical catalysts is energy consuming, leads to undesirable side products, requires expensive wastewater treatment, and makes it difficult to recover the glycerol. Enzymatic production of biodiesel omits these difficulties and is workable at milder conditions. It is not economical when an enzyme is used in free form, which makes the recovery of the enzyme impossible. Immobilization not only increases the stability of enzyme, also favours to use the enzyme several times thereby reducing the production cost.

Transesterification of palm oil with methanol was carried out by lipase PS from *Burkholderia cepacia*. In order to save the cost of the enzyme, lipase PS was further used in immobilized form. Selection of suitable immobilization matrix and techniques is important to ensure effective usage of enzyme and sustainability. Lipase from *Burkholderia cepacia* was encapsulated in κ-carrageenan by co-extrusion method forming a liquid core capsule with a diameter ranging 1.3–1.8 mm. The encapsulated lipase showed good pH, temperature, and storage stability similar to free lipase and retains 72.3 % of its original activity after using for 6 cycles. The K_m and V_{max} values were similar to that of free lipase. *Burkholderia cepacia* lipase encapsulated in κ-carrageenan showed good stability in various alcohols and alkenes and the encapsulated lipase could be stored at room temperature for 10 days without significant change to its activity.

The biodiesel production using encapsulated lipase was carried out in the stirred tank and packed bed batch reactor. The results revealed that stirred tank batch reactor shows higher methyl ester conversion compared to the packed bed reactor for the same set of reaction conditions. At optimized reaction conditions, 1:7 oil/methanol molar ratio, 1 g water, 5.25 g immobilized lipase, 72 h reaction time and 23.7 g relative centrifugal force, methyl ester conversion of up to 100 % was achieved in transesterification of palm oil using the encapsulated lipase in stirred tank reactor. The immobilized lipase also proved to be stable and lost little activity when subjected to repeated uses. From the experimental studies the kinetics parameters K_m and V_{max} were determined to be $K_m = 600$ (mol/m³) $V_{max} = 0.84$ (mol/m³.Min). Using the kinetics parameters the model equation for biodiesel production using encapsulated lipase in stirred tank bioreactor was derived. When the initial concentration of substrate and the desired conversions are known, the required batch time t can thus easily be calculated using the model equation.

The economic assessment of biodiesel production using immobilized enzyme catalyst process was challenging compared to the current alkali process. However, The LCA studies showed that biodiesel production using immobilized enzyme catalyst has lesser impact on the environment compared to the alkali catalyst and soluble enzyme catalyst. Thus κ-carrageenen encapsulated lipase could be a potential immobilized enzyme for ecofriendly production of biodiesel.

References

Akoh CC, Chang SS, Lee GG, Shaw JJ (2007) Enzymatic approach to biodiesel production. J Agri Food Chem 55:8995–9005

Alejandro GM (2003) Enzyme kinetics: a modern approach. John Wiley & Sons, New York

Al-Zuhair S (2005) Production of biodiesel by lipase-catalyzed transesterification of vegetable oils: a kinetics study. Biotechnol Prog 21:1442–1448

Anita A, Sastry CA, Hashim MA (1997) Immobilization of urease in vermiculite. Bioprocess Biosyst Eng 16:375–380

Bayramoğlu G, Kaya B, Arıca MY (2005) Immobilization of Candida rugosa lipase onto spacer-arm attached poly(GMA-HEMA-EGDMA) microspheres. Food Chem 92:261–268

Betigeri SS, Neau SH (2002) Immobilization of lipase using hydrophilic polymers in the form of beads. Biomaterials 23:3627–3636

Brandenberger H, Widmer F (1997) A new multi-nozzle encapsulation immobilization system to produce uniform beads of alginate. J Biotechnol 63:73–80

Cao L (2005) Immobilized enzymes: science or art? Curr Opin Chem Biol 9:217–226

Chen J, Liu M, Jin S, Liu H (2008) Synthesis and characterization of κ-carrageenan/poly(N, N-diethylacrylamide) semi-interpenetrating polymer network hydrogels with rapid response to temperature. Polym Adv Technol 19:1656–1663

De Queiroz AA, Passos DE, De Brito AS, Gerald SS, Higa OZ, Michele V (2006) Alginate-poly(vinyl alcohol) core- shell microspheres for lipase immobilization. J Appl Polym Sci 102:1553–1560

Dizge N, Keskinlera B, Tanrisevenb A (2008) Covalent attachment of microbial lipase onto micro-porous styrene–divinylbenzene copolymer by means of polyglutaraldehyde. Colloids Surf B Biointerfaces 66:34–38

Dizge N, Aydiner C, Derya YI, Mahmut B, Aziz T, Keskinler B (2009) Biodiesel production from sunflower, soybean, and waste cooking oils by transesterification using lipase immobilized onto a novel microporous polymer. Bioresour Technol 100:1983–1991

Dossat V, Combes D, Marty A (2002) Lipase-catalyzed transesterification of high oleic sunflower oil. Enzyme Microb Technol 30:90–94

Du W, Xu Y, Liu D, Li Z (2005) Study on acyl migration in immobilized lipozyme TL-catalyzed transesterification of soybean oil for biodiesel production. J Mol Catal B: Enzym 37:68–71

Griffiths PC, Stilbs P, Yu GE, Booth C (1995) Role of molecular architecture in polymer diffusion: a PGSE-NMR study of linear and cyclic poly(ethylene oxide). J Phys Chem 99:16752–16756

Halim SFA, Kamaruddin AH (2008) Catalytic studies of lipase on FAME production from waste cooking palm oil in a tert-butanol system. Process Biochem 43:1436–1439

Halim SFA, Kamaruddin AH, Fernando WJN (2009) Continuous biosynthesis of biodiesel from waste cooking palm oil in a packed bed reactor: optimization using response surface methodology (RSM) and mass transfer studies. Bioresour Technol 100:710–716

Harding KG, Dennis JS, Blottnitz HV, Harrison STL (2008) A life-cycle comparison between inor-ganic and biological catalysis for the production of biodiesel. J Cleaner Prod 16:1368–1378

Hsu A, Jones K, Marmer WN, Foglia TA (2001) Production of alkyl esters from tallow and grease using lipase immobilized in a phyllosilicate sol-gel. J Am oil Chem Soc 78:585–588

Hung TC, Giridhar R, Chiou SH, Wu WT (2003) Binary immobilization of Candida rugosa lipase on chitosan. J Mol Catal B: Enzym 26:69–78

Iso M, Chen B, Eguchi M, Kudo T, Shrestha S (2001) Production of biodiesel fuel from triglycer-ides and alcohol using immobilized lipase. J Mol Catal B: Enzym 16:53–58

Jegannathan KR, Abang S, Poncelet D, Chan ES, Ravindra P (2008) Production of biodiesel using immobilized lipase- a critical review. Crit Rev Biotechnol 28:253–264

Jegannathan KR, Chan ES, Ravindra P (2009) Physical and stability characteristics of Burkholderia cepacia lipase encapsulated in κ-carrageenan. J Mol Catal B: Enzym 58:78–83

Jegannathan KR, Leong JY, Chan ES, Ravindra P (2010) Production of biodiesel from palm oil using liquid core lipase encapsulated in κ-carrageenan. Fuel 89:2272–2277

Jegannathan KR, Chan ES, Ravindra P (2011a) Economic assessment for the production of biodiesel from palm oil using alkali catalysts, soluble enzyme catalysts and immobilized enzyme catalyst. Renew Sustain Energy Rev 15:745–751

Jegannathan KR, Chan ES, Ravindra P (2011b) Life cycle assessment of biodiesel production using alkali, soluble and immobilized enzyme catalyst processes. Biomass Bioenergy 35:4221–4422

Kaieda M, Samukawa T, Kondo A, Fukuda H (2001) Effect of methanol and water contents on production of biodiesel Fuel from plant oil catalyzed by various lipases in a solvent-free system. J Biosci Bioeng 91:12–15

Kayode Coker A (2001) Modeling of chemical kinetics and reactor design. Gulf Publishing Company, Houston

Kılınç A, Teke M, Önal S, Telefoncu A (2006) Immobilization of pancreatic lipase on chitin and chitosan. Prep Biochem Biotechnol 36:153–163

Kumari V, Shah S, Gupta MN (2007) Preparation of biodiesel by lipase-catalyzed transesterification of high free fatty acid containing oil from Madhuca indica. Energy Fuel 21:368–372

Li L, Du W, Liu D, Wang L, Li Z (2006) Lipase catalyzed transesterification of rapeseed oils for biodiesel production with a novel organic solvents as the reaction medium. J Mol Catal B: Enzym 43:58–62

Lu J, Nie K, Xie F, Wang F, Tan T (2007) Enzymatic synthesis of fatty acids methyl esters from lard with immobilized Candida sp. 99–125. Process Biochem 42:1367–1370

Macario A, Moliner M, Corma A, Giordano G (2009) Increasing stability and productivity of lipase enzyme by encapsulation in a porous organic–inorganic system. Micropor Mesopor Mat 118:334–340

Mittelbach M (1990) Lipase catalyzed alcoholysis of sunflower oil. J Am Oil Chem Soc 67: 168–170

Munjal N, Sawhney SK (2002) Stability and properties of mushroom tyrosinase entrapped in alginate, polyacrylamide and gelatin gels. Enzyme Microb Technol 30:613–619

Noureddini H, Gao X, Philkana RS (2005) Immobilized Pseudomonas cepacia lipase for biodiesel fuel production from soybean oil. Bioresour Technol 96:769–777

Orcaire O, Buisson P, Pierre AC (2006) Application of silica aerogel encapsulated lipases in the synthesis of biodiesel by transesterification reactions. J Mol Catal B: Enzym 42:106–113

Pencreac'h G, Leullier M, Baratti JC (1997) Properties of free and immobilized lipase from Pseudomonas cepacia. Biotechnol Bioeng 56:181–189

Rayon D, Daz M, Ellenrieder G, Locatelli S (2007) Enzymatic production of biodiesel from cotton seed oil using t-butanol as a solvent. Bioresour Technol 98:648–653

Salis A, Pinna M, Monduzzi M, Solinas V (2005) Biodiesel production from triolein and short chain alcohols through biocatalysis. J Biotechnol 119:291–299

Samukawa T, Kaieda M, Matsumoto T, Ban K, Kondo A, Shimada Y, Noda H, Fukuda H (2000) Pretreatment of immobilized Candida Antarctica lipase for biodiesel fuel production from plant oil. J Biosci Bioeng 90:180–183

Sankalia MG, Mashru RC, Sankalia MJ, Sutariya VB (2006) Stability improvement of alpha-amylase entrapped in kappa-carrageenan beads: Physicochemical characterization and optimization using composite index. Int J Pharm 312:1–14

Schuler ML, Kargi F (1992) Bioprocess engineering – basic concepts. Prentice-Hall, New Jersy

Shah S, Gupta MN (2006) Lipase catalyzed preparation of biodiesel from Jatropha oil in a solvent free system. Process Biochem 42:409–414

Shah S, Sharma A, Gupta MN (2004) Biodiesel preparation by lipase-catalyzed transesterification of Jatropha oil. Energy Fuel 18:154–159

Soumanou MM, Bornscheuer UT (2003) Improvement in lipase-catalyzed synthesis of fatty acid methyl esters from sunflower oil. Enzyme Microb Technol 33:97–103

Sung HH, Lan MN, Lee SN, Hwang SM, Koo YM (2007) Lipase-catalyzed biodiesel production from soybean oil in ionic liquids. Enzyme Microb Technol 41:480–483

Tang ZX, Qian JQ, Shi LE (2007) Characterizations of immobilized neutral lipase on chitosan nano-particles. Mater Lett 61:37–40

Toreki W, Manukian A, Strohschein R (2004) Hydrocapsules and method of preparation thereof. US Patent 6,780,507

Tosa T, Sato T, Mori T, Yamamoto K, Takata I, Nishida Y, Chibata I (1979) Immobilization of enzymes and microbial cells using carrageenan as matrix. Biotechnol Bioeng 21:1697–1709

Tumturk H, Karaca N, Demirel G, Sahin F (2007) Preparation and application of poly(N, N-dimethylacrylamide-co-acrylamide) and poly(N-isopropylacrylamide-co-acrylamide)/κ--carrageenan hydrogels for immobilization of lipase. Int J Biol Macromol 40:281–285

Vrushali D, Hareshkumar K, Datta M (2009) Ethyl isovalerate synthesis using Candida rugosa lipase immobilized on silica nanoparticles prepared in nonionic reverse micelles. Process Biochem 44:349–352

Wang L, Du W, Liu D, Li L, Dai N (2006) Lipase-catalyzed biodiesel production from soybean oil deodorizer distillate with absorbent present in tert-butanol system. J Mol Catal B: Enzym 43:29–32

Watanabe Y, Shimada Y, Sugihara A, Noda H, Fukuda H, Tominaga Y (2000) Continuous production of biodiesel fuel from vegetable oil using immobilized Candida antarctica Lipase. J Am Oil Chem Soc 77:355–360

Watanabe Y, Shimada Y, Sugihara A, Tominaga Y (2001) Enzymatic conversion of waste edible oil to biodiesel fuel in a fixed-bed bioreactor. J Am Oil Chem Soc 78:703–707

Winston J P, Miskiel FJ, Valli RC (1994) Composition and process for gelatin-free soft capsules. US Patent 5342626

Xu Y, Du W, Liu D (2005) Study on the kinetics of enzymatic interesterification of triglycerides for biodiesel production with methyl acetate as the acyl acceptor. J Mol Catal B: Enzym 32: 241–245

Yadav GD, Jadhav SR (2005) Synthesis of reusable lipases by immobilization on hexagonal mesoporous silica and encapsulation in calcium alginate: transesterification in non-aqueous medium. Micropor Mesopor Mat 86:215–222

Yagiz F, Kazan D, Akin AN (2007) Biodiesel production from waste oils by using lipase immobilized on hydrotalcite and zeolites. Chem Eng J 134:262–267

Yang G, Tian-Wei T, Kai-Li N, Fang W (2006) Immobilization of lipase on macroporous resin and its application in synthesis of biodiesel in low aqueous media. Chin J Biotechnol 22:114–118

Zeng HG, Liao K, Deng X, Jiang H, Zhang F (2009) Characterization of the lipase immobilized on Mg–Al hydrotalcite for biodiesel. Process Biochem 44:791–798

Zhang GQ, Zha LS, Zhou MH, Ma JH, Liang BR (2005) Rapid deswelling of sodium alginate/poly(N-isopropylacrylamide) semi-interpenetrating polymer network hydrogels in response to temperature and pH changes. Colloids Polym Sci 283:431–438

Nomenclature

r	Radius, m
K	Boltzmann constant kg m^2/s^2
T	Temperature K
t	Time h
E	Activation energy, J/mol
R	Gas constant = 8.314 J/mol °K
V	Reaction rate constant or velocity constant
De	Diffusivity m^2/s
r	Particle radius m
V$''m$	Maximum reaction rate mol/m^3 sec (transeserification)
V$'$max	Maximum reaction rate (U/mg-protein) (hydrolysis)
K$'$m	Michalis Menton constant (mM) (hydrolysis)
km	Michalis Menton constant mol/ m^3 (transeserification)
C$_S$	Concentration of the substrate at time t
C$_{SO}$	Concentration of the substrate at time $t =0$
V$_o$	Frequency factor or pre-exponential factor
+r$_p$	Rate of product formation (Methyl esters)
−r$_s$	Rate of disappearance of S (Triglycerides)
A$_{410nm}$	Absorbance at 410 nm
Δε	Molar extinction of nitrophenol
η	Effectiveness factor
Φ	Thiele modulus
β	Michalis constant dimensionless number

© The Author(s) 2015
P. Ravindra, K.R. Jegannathan, *Production of biodiesel using lipase encapsulated in κ-carrageenan*, SpringerBriefs in Bioengineering, DOI 10.1007/978-3-319-10822-3